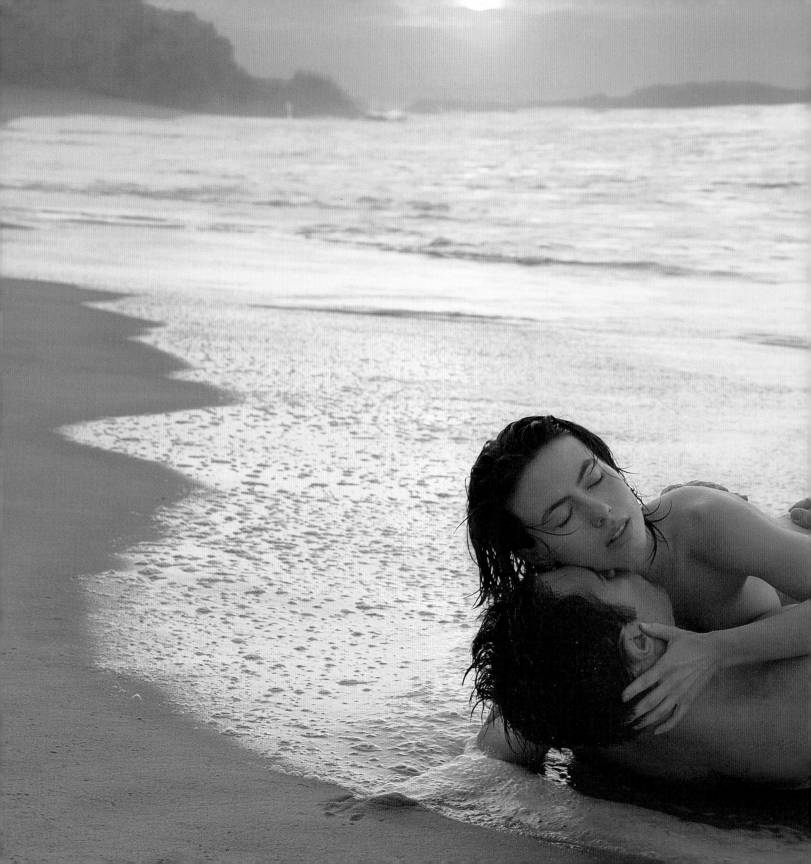

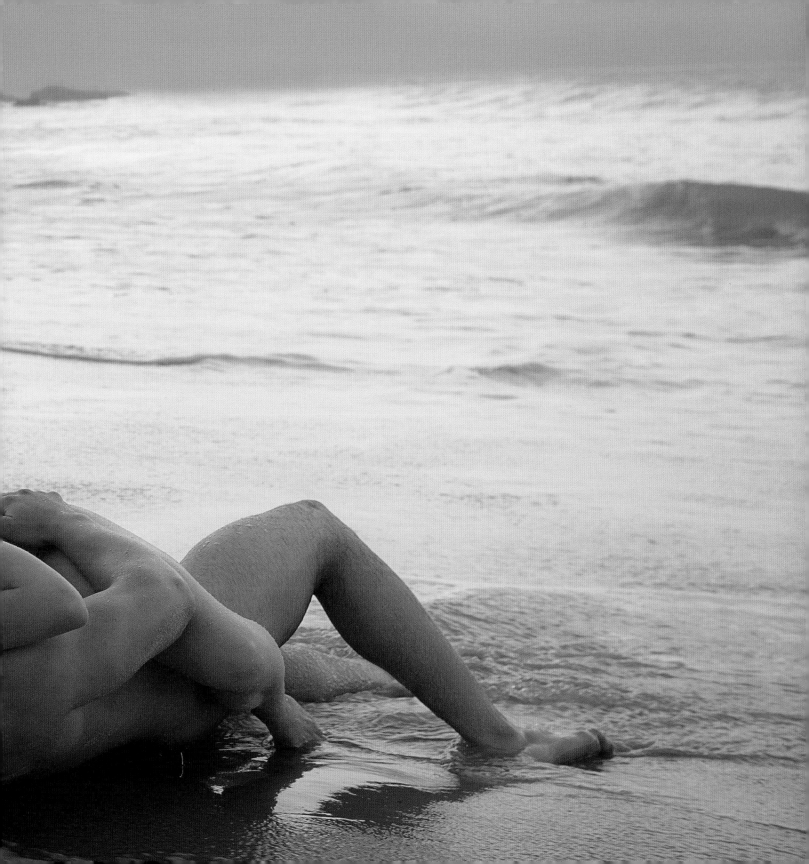

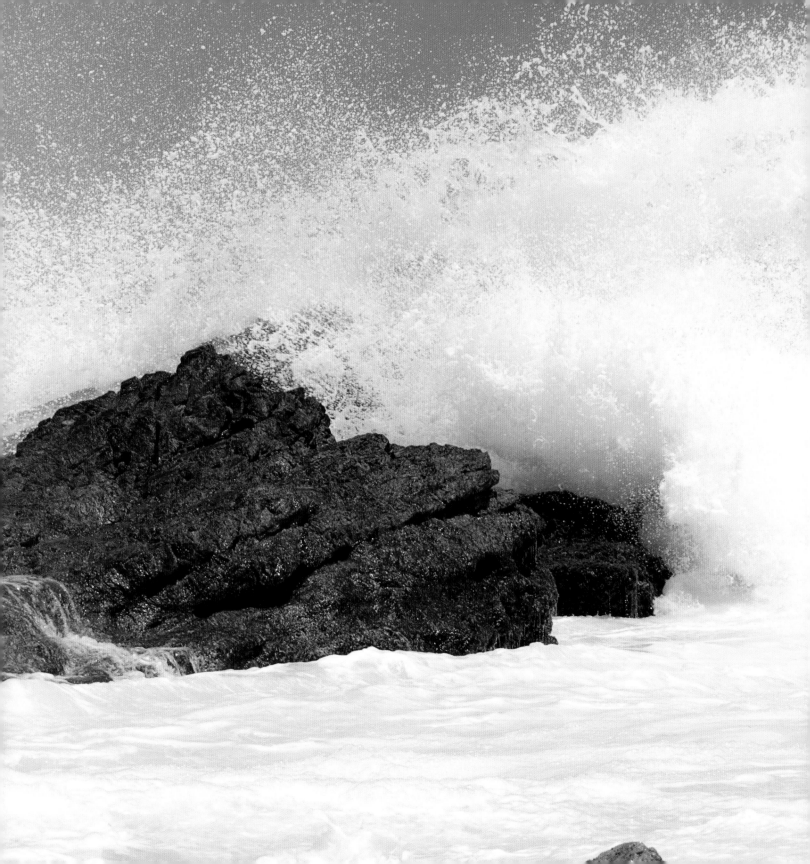

WET

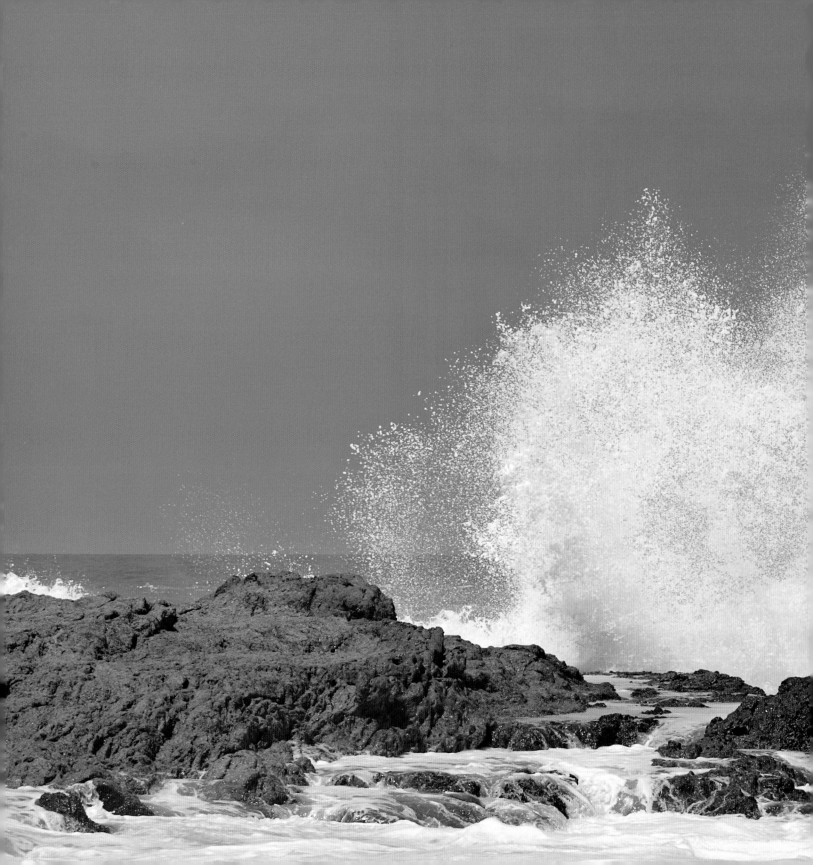

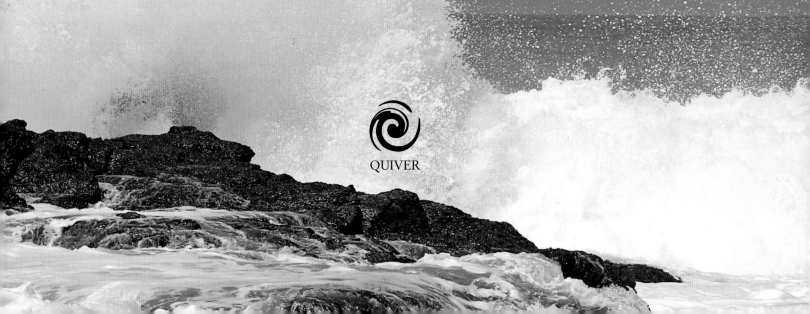

WET

EROTIC ADVENTURES IN WATER

QUIVER

First published in the USA in 2007 by
Quiver, a member of
Quayside Publishing Group
33 Commercial Street
Gloucester, MA 01930

11 10 09 08 07   1 2 3 4 5

ISBN-13: 978-1-59233-257-1
ISBN-10: 1-59233-257-9

Library of Congress Cataloging-in-Publication Data
Kate, Ellen.
  Wet : erotic adventures in water / Ellen Kate.
    p. cm.
  ISBN-13: 978-1-59233-257-1
  ISBN-10: 1-59233-257-9
  1. Water sex. 2. Sex instruction. I. Title.
    HQ31.K373 2007
    613.9'6--dc22

2006100325

Cover design by Michael Brock
Book design by Rachel Fitzgibbon
Photography by Allan Penn Photography

Printed and bound in Singapore

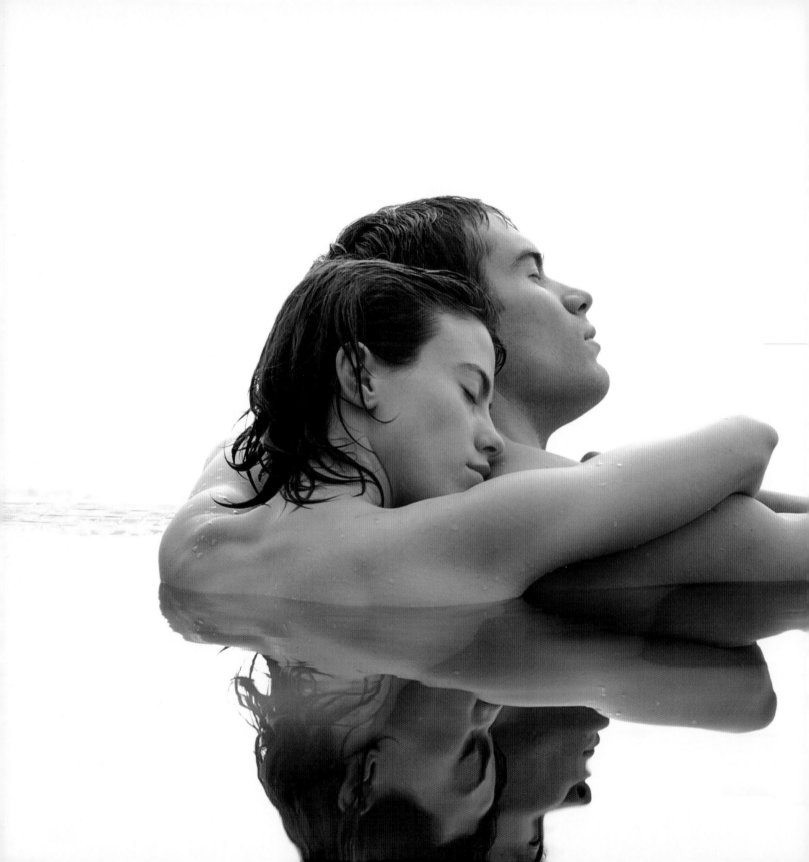

INTRODUCTION
Aqua Erotica

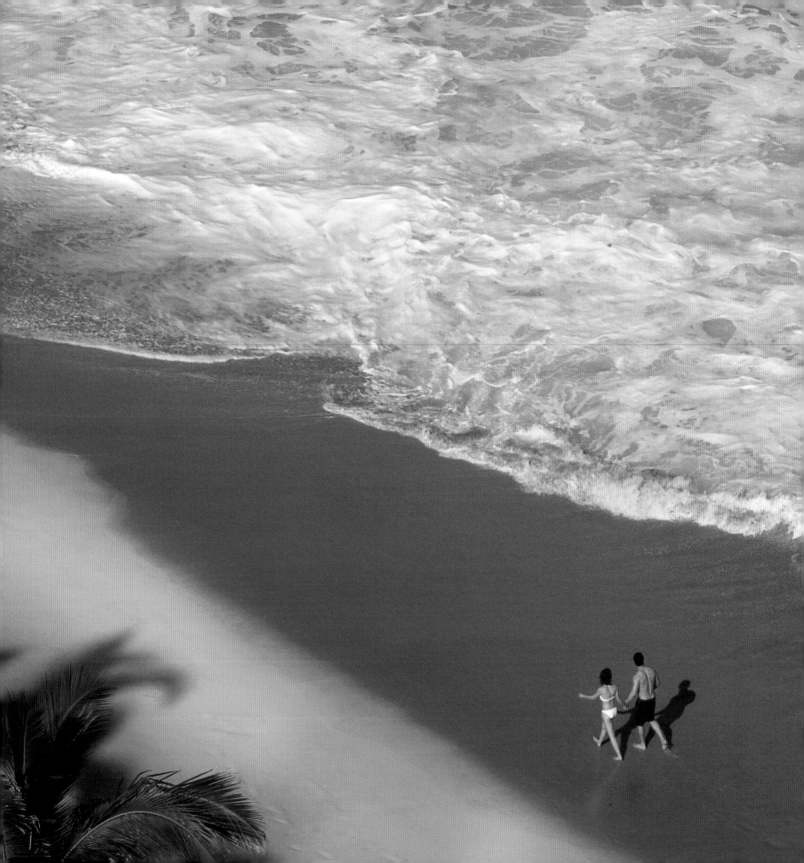

INTRODUCTION

*P*OLL ANY NUMBER OF PEOPLE about what they find hot, and chances are that someone will mention water. You are apt to hear about turn-ons such as sex on the beach, wet t-shirts, hot tubs, waterbeds, massage oil, shower sex, ice cubes, bubble baths, underwater encounters, rain, waterfalls, and oral sex. Individually, these turn-ons don't necessarily stand out. But when all of these ideas are combined, it becomes clear that a lot of people find wetness incredibly exciting!

The effect water has on everything from aesthetics to sensation is amazingly varied and appeals to many instincts. Aquatic sex is just as likely to be playful, sexy, and exciting as it is to be tender and intimate. By itself, water is eternally pure, but it can easily be incorporated into naughtier endeavors without too much effort. For instance, sex in a hot tub while sipping martinis might seem like a delightfully saucy experience. Making love on a moonlit beach can be the height of romance. An underwater striptease game can be silly and playful. Dressing up as a pirate and acting out your kidnap fantasy could be a way to channel more nautical desires. Though at first glance each of these experiences seem worlds apart, when we recognize water's role in all of them, it becomes easier to understand that this liquid element, more than any other, appeals to countless erotic impulses.

Explore the Possibilities

Regardless of whether you are coupled, single, kinky, or conservative, aqueous sex play can deliver in a way that nothing else can. *Wet* provides a forum to showcase the extreme variety of sexual possibilities afforded by this expression of sexuality. But *Wet* is not simply some sociological study of the human animal. It is also a super steamy read! Water enthusiasts will expose their raciest fantasies and experiences, and you'll be treated to explicit instructions for sexual techniques as well as detailed descriptions (and depictions) of incredibly wet and wild sex play. *Wet* takes you on an erotic adventure you will not soon forget. Chapter 1, "Diving In," introduces the historical relationship between water and sexuality and explains how each of your five senses can be tantalized in wet ways. In Chapter 2, "Aquatic Arousal," you'll take a journey through wet-inspired arousal. It provides tips for turn-ons and useful advice about the best tools of the trade for sexy fun in the water. Chapter 3, "Positions, Places, and Pleasure," offers information on the hottest sex positions to use in aquatic locations, such as pools, hot tubs, oceans, bathtubs, and showers. You'll even learn new ways to set up sessions of liquid love! In Chapter 4, "Solo Sailing," explore the ways in which you can incorporate water into your private, personal exploits. Toys, techniques, and turn-ons are covered. This chapter also dispels the stigmas that are associated with self-love and explains the health benefits of pleasuring one's self. Chapter 5, "Drying Off," closes the book with a reminder of all the wet ways to enjoy your sexuality. Throughout each chapter, readers are treated to "Wet 'n Wild" tips. These tips are snapshot ideas for enhancing enjoyment in a variety of wet ways. Potential pitfalls are also addressed, and suggestions for games, role-playing activities, and even fantasy fodder are included.

Water, Water Everywhere

The appeal of wetness stems in part from a desire to express the primal nature of sexuality. Water can set the mood, intensify sensual touch, or enhance the aesthetics of one's surroundings. Plenty of people have discovered that having sex in *wet* ways will spice up any erotic encounter. Consider how often water and wet sex are featured in depictions of sexuality: Sweat-drenched models dance in music videos, rain cascades over reunited lovers embracing on the movie screen. And who wouldn't want to buy a soda after watching a steamy hottie quench an incredible thirst in one of the countless advertisements that use the raw power of wetness as a selling point? There's no doubt about it—wherever you look, wet is red hot!

Like water itself, sexuality can be fluid, changing shape over the course of a lifetime. One minute we might contentedly enjoy the kiss of a longtime lover at home in bed, and the next we may crave a sweaty entanglement on the shores of a tropical beach with a perfect stranger. The beauty of exploring the aquatic aspects of sexuality lies in the fact that there are just so many possibilities, and *Wet* speaks to the countless desires we experience. It doesn't matter whether aquatic play is a staple of your sex life or something about which you are simply curious, *Wet* provides plenty of options for exploration and arousal. If you want to spice up your day-to-day sex life, learn hot vacation sex tips, or add an aquatic element to your already sizzling encounters, this book will guide you with the hottest suggestions and ideas for creative new venues and outlets for exploration. So strip down and get ready to dive in!

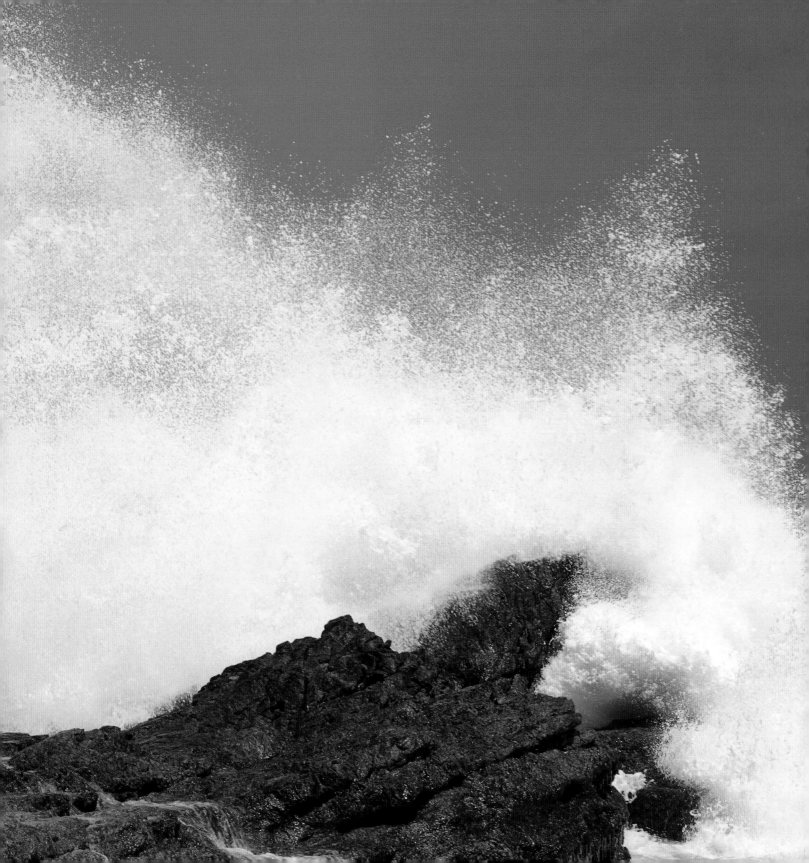

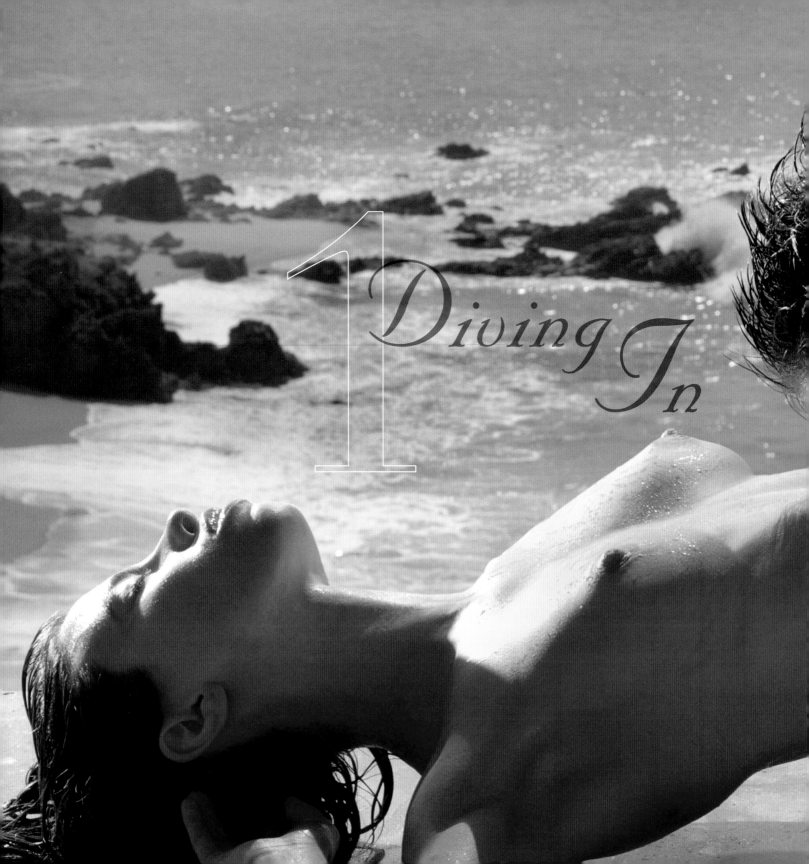

1

Diving In

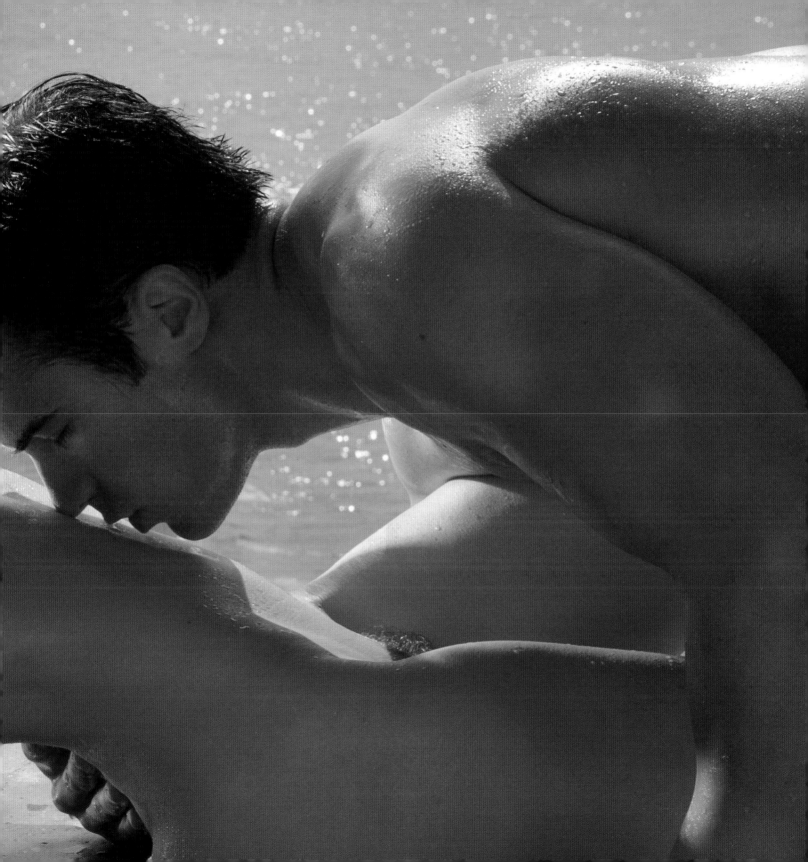

1 Diving In

WHEN IT COMES TO SEX, WETTER IS ALWAYS BETTER. Water is a highly sensual and amazingly versatile fluid, and as a result, wet sex can be sweaty and raw or pure and innocent. As the source of all life, water has the power to sustain us. It is the basis of our evolutionary origins, the quencher of insatiable thirst, and a tangible reminder of the sexual juices we produce during arousal. The ardor that emerges underwater, on island vacations, or standing under one's own shower is a liquid lust that can be channeled into countless forms of sexual expression. Making sex play wet, be it by soaking yourself, finding an aquatic venue, or acting out a water-themed fantasy, is just about the hottest way to spice up any sexual encounter.

But what's so great about wetness?

Much like fish, which instinctively swim toward a glittering lure bobbing in the water, humans are attracted to sparkly things. Dangling diamond earrings, flashing sequins, and even the gleam of a shining white smile, are all tantalizing suggestions of wetness that hint at our base instincts. But why do we find wetness so appealing in the first place? One reason is because shimmering water just makes everything look better. Many cinematographers water down their sets, even if the scene is not intended to be a rainy one, in order to capture the play of light off a slick surface. Fashion models are spritzed during photo shoots to highlight everything from cleavage to the glint of a bracelet encircling a slim wrist. Wetness adds pizzazz and glamour and makes the mundane a little more enticing.

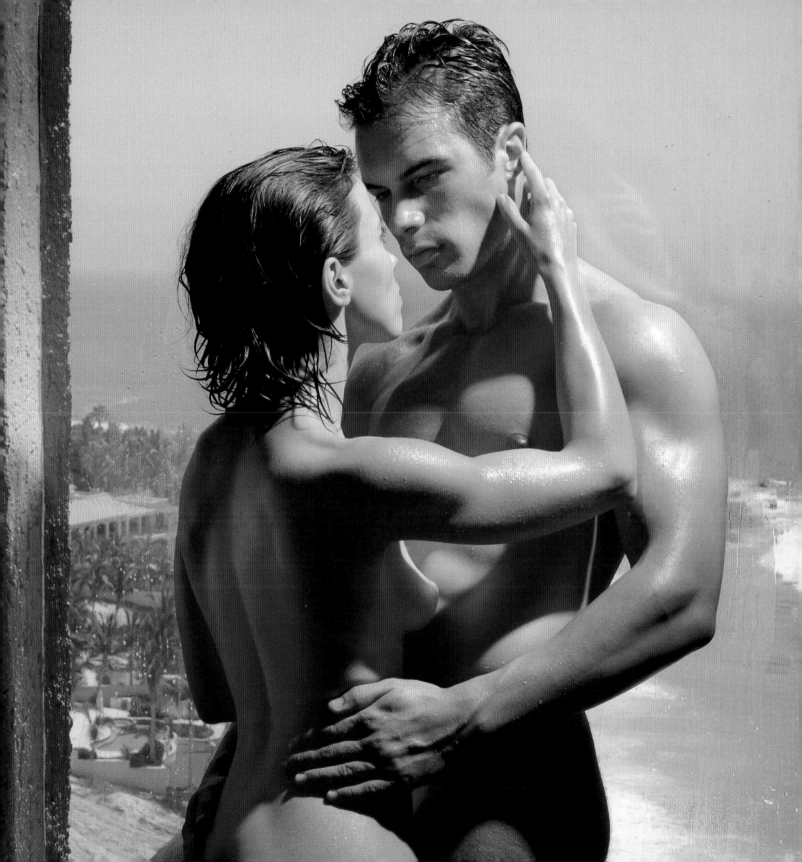

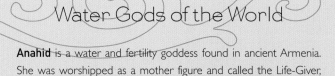

Water Gods of the World

Anahid is a water and fertility goddess found in ancient Armenia. She was worshipped as a mother figure and called the Life-Giver, Golden Mother, and Benefactress of All Mankind.

In Greek mythology, **Aphrodite** is the goddess of love, beauty, and sexual pleasure. She was born when Cronus castrated his father, Uranus, and threw his genitals into the ocean. Out of this Aphrodite arose. She was worshipped by many and had devoted priestesses. Having sex with these priestesses was considered a method of worship.

The **Apsaras** were beautiful Indian nature spirits and water nymphs. The Apsaras would dance and perform for the gods in their palaces and were seen as the inspirations for love. At times they were sent to tempt rishis, or Brahmans, who were supposed to abstain from carnal pleasures.

Benten originated as a Japanese sea and water goddess. Her powers expanded and she became the goddess of love, eloquence, wisdom, the arts, music, knowledge, good fortune, and water. She is the patroness of geishas, dancers, and musicians.

In Greek mythology, **Naiads**, **Nereids**, and **Oceanids** were nymphs who lounged in bodies of water. Described as young and beautiful, these nymphs were famous for luring men into romantic entanglements.

Poseidon, the god of the sea, used his powers to seduce women and project his virility. He had countless love affairs and fathered numerous children. Poseidon married many times, including to a Nereid with whom he fathered **Triton**. Triton, half-human, half-fish, rode the waves on horses and sea monsters carrying a twisted conch shell, which he blows either violently or gently, to stir up or calm the waves.

Also from Greek mythology, the **Sirens** were creatures with the head of a female and the body of a bird. They lured mariners to their destruction on the rocks surrounding their island with the irresistible charm of their song.

When it comes to sex, water has an arousing effect for many people. A scenic lake setting can quickly turn into the site of a passionate sexcapade. A shower stall can effortlessly transform into a hot lovemaking venue. Even an innocent glass of water can hold immense appeal if sipped by the right lips. Much of the appeal of wetness stems from a desire to express the primal nature of sexuality. Slick bodies sliding across each other demonstrate daring, abandon, and passion. As a result, many people find liquid in all its various forms intensely arousing.

"Wet is sexy," says Mike, 33. "Someone who is willing to get soaking wet during sex seems less inhibited than someone who always wants to stay dry. Being wet is dangerous and exciting." Allison takes this view further. "Having sex in the water seems natural and spiritual and helps me feel like I am engaging in a sacred act. I also love the idea of rolling around naked in the rain and mud." Anderson, 28, sees water as a life-giving element and likes to bring that into his sex play. "Water sustains us, and sex perpetuates us. The combination to me is a reaffirmation of the life-cycle."

Other people simply find wetness sexy in and of itself. "I like to see a woman's nipples showing under a wet bra or shirt," says Bram, 22, a fan of water-themed porn. Dominique, 18, gets excited reading steamy tales involving liquid love. "I'm into erotica that has to do with water and oceans. I must have reread a few of the same stories a hundred times imagining how I would recreate scenes one day." Getting wet is one of the simplest ways to heat up a sexual encounter. Nothing else is a better conduit for the countless forms of sexual expression that we are capable of.

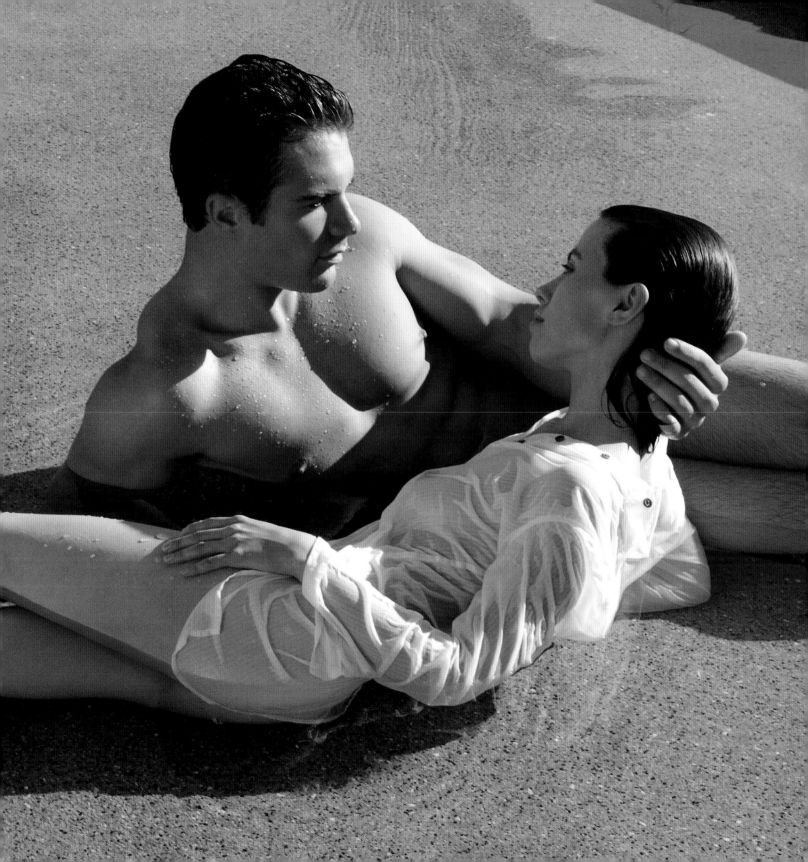

A Little History

It should come as no surprise that the association of water with sexuality is ancient and universal, highlighting the deeply ingrained relationship between sexuality and the life force itself. Almost every culture has a creation story, a fertility tale, or a love god or goddess whose powers are yielded through an aquatic connection. In fact, many of these ancient associations continue to influence our contemporary understanding of sexuality. A scantily clad woman standing near the water's edge is a vision many find alluring today. It is also one that has been used to sell everything from shampoo to island vacations, and it is by no means an invention of our modern era. Similar images can actually be traced back to some of the earliest cultures. For example, the ancients Greeks often paired images of young women with water. Greeks were particularly fond of depictions of naiads, fresh-water nymphs who inhabited springs and lakes, lounging semi-clothed by the water's edge, and they often used these to represent sexuality or desire.

The Mythical Mermaid

One of the most enduring images to capture the true sensuality of wetness is the mermaid. Almost all cultures tell tales of mermaids and mermen who inhabit the ocean depths. Mermaids are wet, bare-breasted, and youthful. They wear seductive smiles and sing tantalizing songs. They are mythical and mysterious and utterly unattainable. This, of course, is part of what makes them so incredibly enticing. The sexuality of the mermaid has been a constant tease throughout history: Sailors have long told tales of these exotic creatures, artists have sculpted their form, and fairy tales the world over (as well as contemporary films like 1984's *Splash*) hold our imagination by describing mermaids who are torn between land loves and aquatic immortality. Recently, mermaids even entered the realm of erotic films. A quick Internet search turns up porn with titles such as *Mermaid Fantasy, Mermaids-Flesh, Sea & Symphony,* and hard-core take-offs on the Disney film *The Little Mermaid. Teenage Mermaid Fanta-sea*, a film

by sex pioneer and self-described "post-porn modernist" Annie Sprinkle, also attempts to capture the sexual allure of the mermaid. In her film, Annie plays an older mermaid who initiates a young teenage mermaid into the discovery of her sexuality with the help of a sexy merman, and in the process touches on the many levels of mermaid appeal.

A Contemporary Mermaid

Marigny Lee swam as a professional mermaid at New York City's Coral Room bar. Every night she would slide into her tail and splash into an enormous tank that sat behind the bar. There, in her shell bikini top and mermaid tail, she would twist and twirl among fish and seaweed, treating patrons to a live mermaid show. Marigny believes her appeal was in the tease.

"As a mermaid I would flirt shamelessly though the tank, blowing kisses and flipping my hair at the men who crowded around," she says. "When I was in my tail, I was sexy and flowing and slippery. Strippers also create a fantasy, but that is more clearly sexual… Mermaids are half-dressed, but despite the fact that we are nearly naked, we are innocent—because that is just how we are supposed to look. And because we are innocent, we are allowed to flirt without taking it any further."

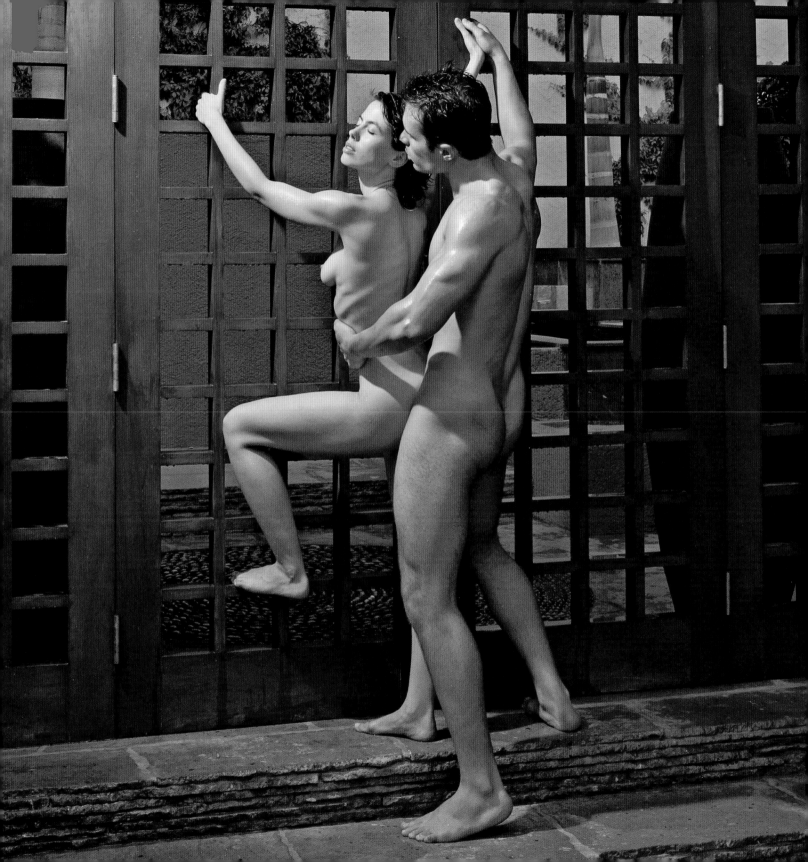

"My girlfriend gave me the most *exotic experience* the other night—she put an ice cube in her mouth and slowly dragged it along *every part of my body*—my abdomen, my nipples, my chest. When she got to my penis, she rubbed it over it, but then immediately put me inside her warm mouth. The sensations were so *mindblowing* that she made me climax before we even had sex!"

—Patrick, 27

The Five Senses

Our senses of smell, taste, touch, sight, and hearing are all integral parts of the sexual experience. Though we often think of sex as a purely physical act, it is, in fact, one that incorporates multiple simultaneous experiences—not all of them tactile. Smells, sounds, and sights can just as easily trigger arousal as can direct touch. Following are a variety of aqueous ideas for arousing each of your senses and awaking feelings that may have otherwise been slumbering.

Taste

Tasting a lover's body for the first time can be extremely exciting, and using your mouth to lick, suck, and tickle is a key part of sex play. Licking something deliciously wet and edible from your lover's body combines the excitement of sex play with the tastiness of your favorite treat. Dribble brandy or cognac over your lover's nipples or navel and then use your tongue to trail it between her breasts or down to his genitals. Take a sip of champagne before giving a blow job and let him feel the sensation of hundreds of bubbles popping in your mouth. Get creative with a bottle of chocolate syrup and experience sweetness bursting in your mouth as your ears thrill to the sounds of your lover's squeals and moans.

Touch

Touch is the sense that is most commonly associated with sexuality. The way we touch and are touched is a crucial element in our sexual enjoyment. Yet everyone enjoys this sensation differently. Some people melt over a soft tickle, while others crave a strong caress or forceful thrust. Whatever your pleasure, you can enhance many of these sensations by adding liquid. Try trailing an ice cube up your lover's thighs, or dribble a half-melted Popsicle down her lower back, stopping only to lap up the sticky liquid. You might also want to work each other over with lubrication, massage oil, or simple soap and water.

Sight

Many people are turned-on visually. The clothes we wear, the images to which we are drawn, and even the desire to keep the lights on during sex can quickly trigger a sexual response. It can be incredibly exciting just to watch a lover bathe or even emerge soaking wet from a swimming pool.

The makers of erotic films understand this, and many play up the visual appeal of wetness, featuring glistening bodies writhing in ecstasy, shower scenes, and other aqueous venues, all of which are designed to arouse the body through the eyes. Much of what is sexy about being wet has to do with skin shining with moisture or damp clothes clinging to attractive bodies. Allowing your eyes to feast on these appealing sights is a great way to get in the mood!

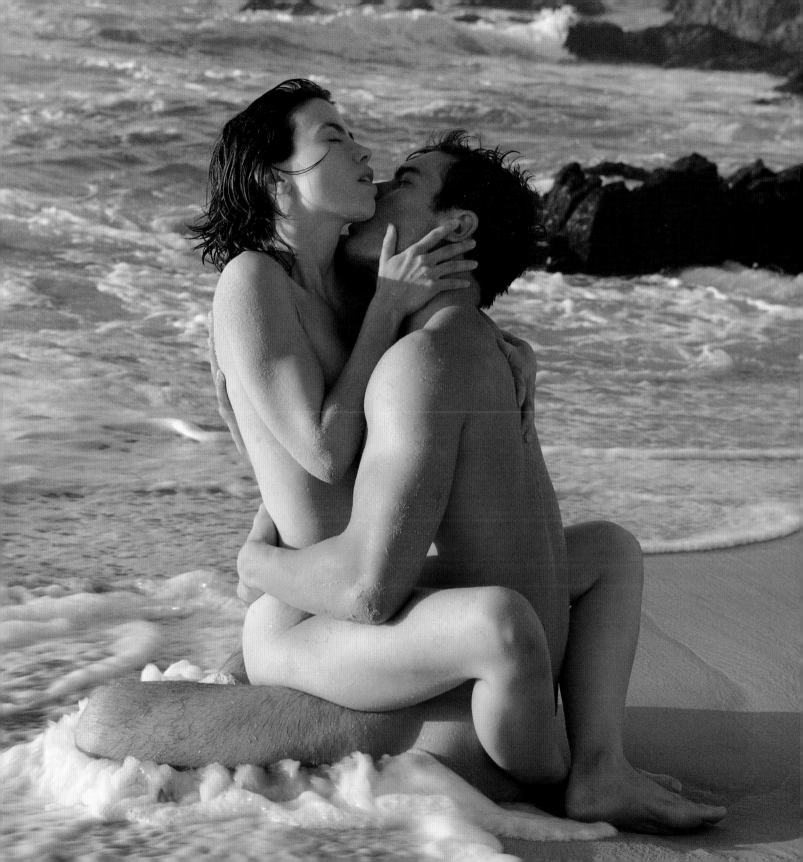

Smell

The olfactory sense often plays an underappreciated role in sexual arousal. Though we frequently try to cover up our natural scents with soaps and perfumes, doing so can mask the pheromones that we send out and the sexual messages they transmit. Our natural muskiness is created by our most intimate body fluids. The scent of sweat, semen, and vaginal secretions are unique to each individual and can awaken a lover's libido like little else. Try shedding the cultural expectations that demand that a lover smell like roses and let yourself enjoy the scents that are actually designed to turn you on. Of course, smells of a less natural variety can also be appealing, and dribbling scented oils into a bath or using them in a massage can create an enticing atmosphere of a slightly less animalistic nature.

Hearing

One of the most exciting parts of sex play is anticipation of what is to come. To keep that anticipation building, read your lover a wet and sexy story from one of the many aquatic themed collections of erotica currently on the market. With titles such as *Aqua Erotica* and *Stories for a Steamy Bath*, you are certain to find a tale that melts your honey into a puddle of desire. Or try talking dirty; you may be pleasantly surprised by how much more exciting sex play can be.

We often try to rush through sex without pausing to fully soak in the entire experience, but taking the time to identify how each of your senses plays a role in sex play can heighten sensation and increase pleasure. Think about setting aside time to focus on each sense. Throw in a few aquatic ideas, and your lover is guaranteed to be delighted by the new adventure.

Just Add Water

When it comes to fantasy fodder and arousal enhancers, there are plenty of options. From foot fetishists to bondage enthusiasts, role players and those who prefer more conventional sex, our preferences are as varied as we are. The beauty of wetness lies in the fact that whatever your passion, almost everything lends itself to a little saturation.

Here are some wet ways to spice up your routine:

- **Nighttime sex in bed before falling asleep:**
  What about starting off with a shower together to get you relaxed and in the mood?

- **Sex back in the hotel after a relaxing day at the beach:**
  Begin your session at a secluded seaside spot before you leave the surf and the sand behind.

- **Making out in your car:**
  Park by a lake or river to let the sounds of the water enhance the mood.

- **Tying up your partner:**
  Fill a bottle with warm water and treat your lover to some well-placed squirts.

- **Presenting your honey with a lingerie fashion show:**
  Spice things up with a wet t-shirt contest you put on for just for one pair of eyes.

When it comes to sex, water is an aphrodisiac that can add a twist to your most intimate encounters!

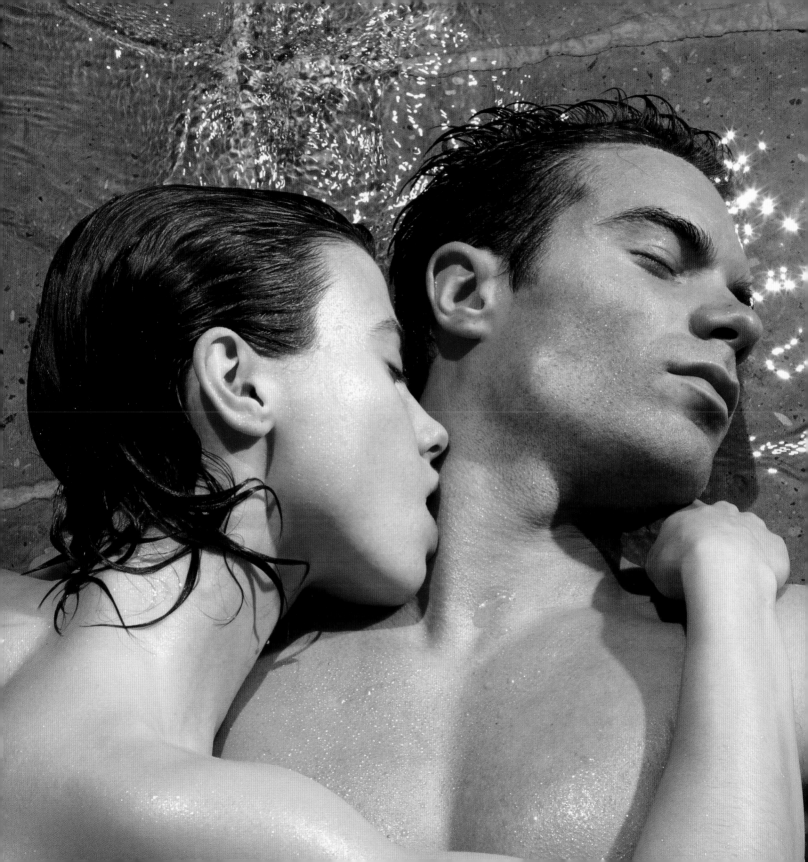

Wet from Head to Toe

Each and every part of the body can enjoy liquid love in a variety of wet and wonderful ways. Bathing and massage are two ways to pamper the body and take advantage of all that the wet stuff has to offer. Set aside a good chunk of time and give your lover a full-body experience. Here's an idea of what your evening could look like:

Start at the bottom and treat your lover to a sensual footbath. If you feel like splurging, invest in a home foot spa. Let your sweetie soak and soothe. Then dry off your honey's toes and work the feet over with a foot massage using your favorite moisturizer. Move your way up the legs for a fully pampering experience. Then lay your lover down for a leisurely massage. Use scented oils to help your hands draw stress from his neck or soothe her tired back.

After the massage, move him into the bathroom for a rinse and explore what the bathtub has to offer. One of the most sensual experiences a couple can share while wet is to bathe together. Washing and soaping up a woman's breasts or a man's chest is a highly erotic experience for both partners. If you have a hand-held shower nozzle, incorporate it to add more liquid luxuriating or bring about amazing aquatic orgasms.

There is no need to stay below the neck. Many people love having their hair professionally washed at a salon. The combination of warm water coursing down your scalp, followed by a relaxing scrub, can be a delicious experience. Just imagine how much more exciting it would be to have your hair lovingly lathered by someone you wouldn't mind jumping into the sack with! Make sure your partner is in a position where is it comfortable to tilt the head back. Then carefully ladle water over her head and rub in shampoo. Be thorough and apply slow, firm pressure to help relieve the tension that is held in the neck and scalp. After the bath, dry off and curl up in bed for a cozy cuddle, or stay damp and enjoy a hot sex session that will require another rinse once you're done.

There are plenty of ways to treat the body to wet and wonderful pleasures. With a little creativity, you're certain to find a way to make every caress a wet one.

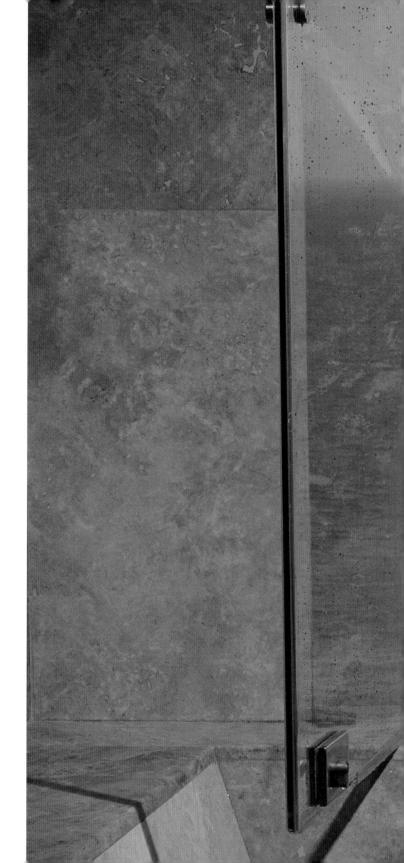

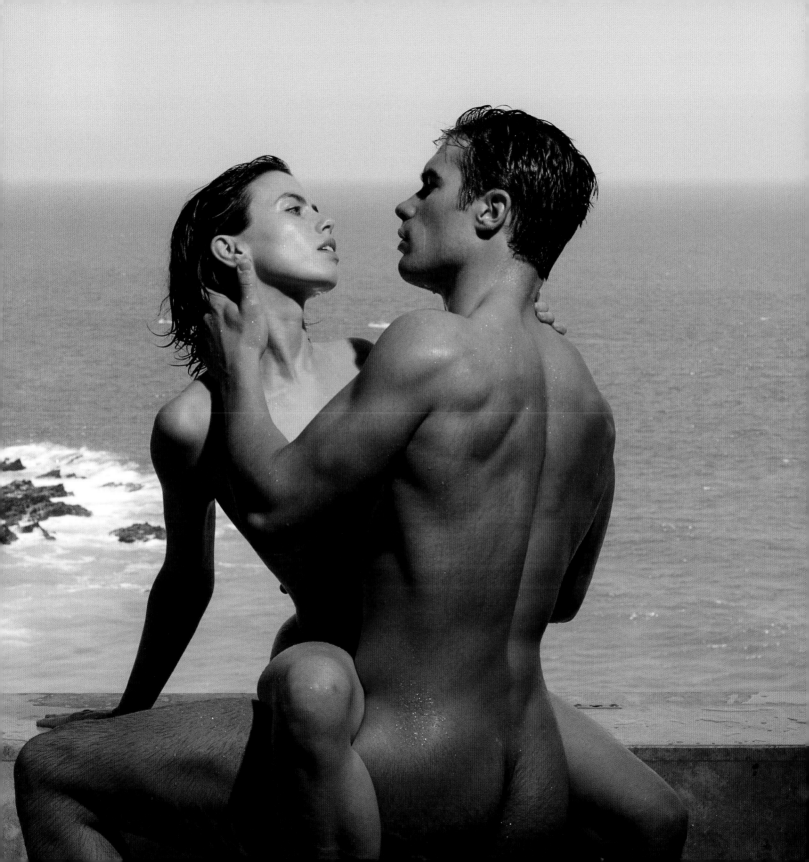

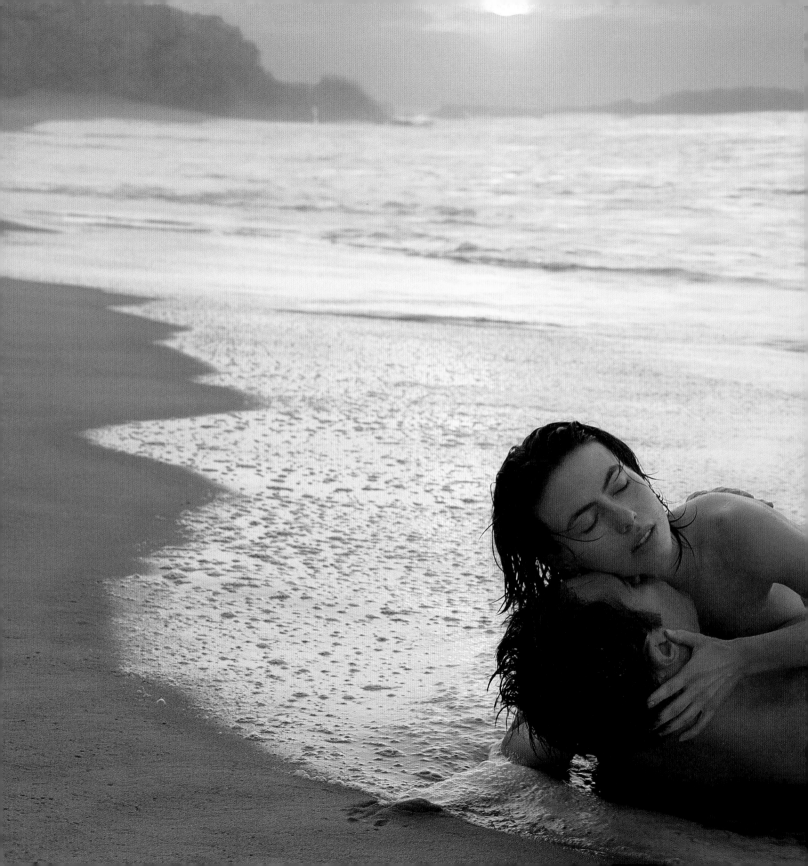

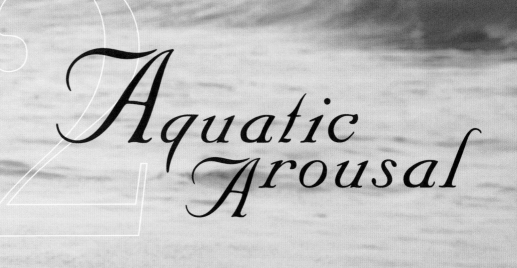

2 Aquatic Arousal

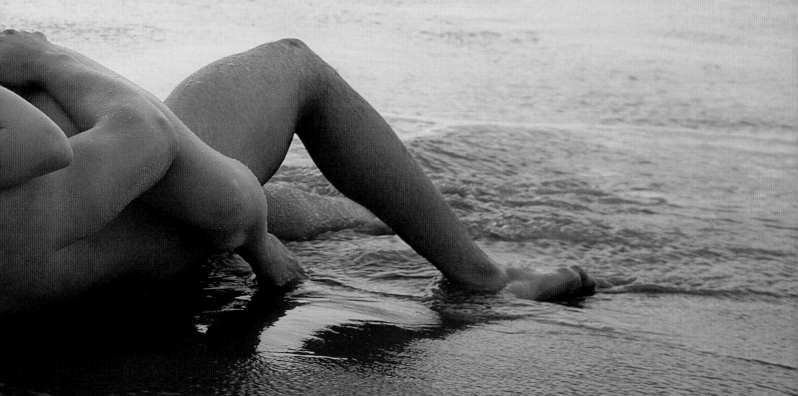

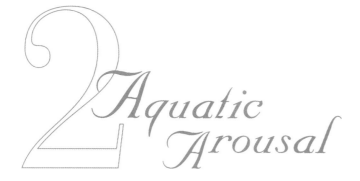

2 Aquatic Arousal

OUR BODIES PRODUCE PLENTY OF FLUIDS, so if you're doing it right, sex is bound to be naturally wet! Once things heat up, we drip sweat, create sexual juices, and swap saliva. It easily follows then, that many of us become aroused by wetness in all its wonderful variations. But the process of arousal is not a cookie-cutter experience; there are plenty of wet ways to enhance every aspect of sex play, from the first kiss to the final climax. Getting there can be half the fun, but being there is pretty amazing too.

Turning On

When it comes to turn-ons, there is no universally agreed-on standard of "sexy." One person can get excited just thinking about a svelte leg donning a stiletto. Another drools over rock-hard abs. A third find her loins burning as she imagines a lusty lover taking her on the dock overlooking a secluded lake.

Rich, 32, explains, "I can be completely unaroused, worrying about my taxes, but if my girl comes out of the shower with wet hair, wrapped in a tiny little towel, everything else I'm thinking about disappears. It's an instant turn-on." Rick doesn't know exactly why this image gets him so excited, but he guesses, "Maybe it's because even though I know she just got out of the shower, seeing her like that makes me think of how she looks when we're having wild, sweaty sex."

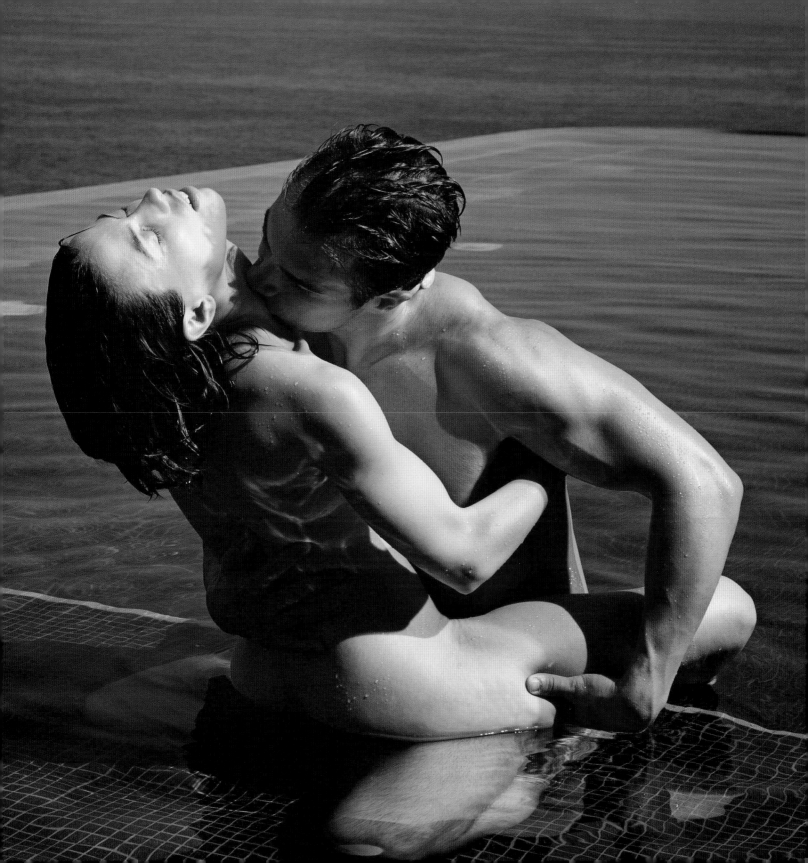

Sheila, 19, uses the power of wetness to get her partner hot and bothered. "I have a really high sex drive. I could have sex every day. Sometimes more than once. My guy is okay doing it once or twice a week. I used to try all these different things to get him in the mood—music, lingerie, porn—but that didn't always work. Once he told me that he loves to watch a woman put on suntan oil. I realized one of the best ways to get him turned on is to let him watch me put on moisturizer! I'll just put on my bathrobe and pick a part of my body and slowly start to work on it. Usually I don't rub it all in because I think he likes when it stays moist and glistening. I'm pretty sure he knows what I'm doing, and he hasn't complained yet."

Venue can also contribute to arousal. Lisa, 31, says, "No matter how hot a guy is, if I walk into his place and there are dirty dishes and underwear on the floor, sex is the last thing I am going to want to do." If the surroundings are less than perfect, turn the focus away from dirty laundry, Lisa suggests. "I'm into romance. Run me a bath and surround the tub with candles. That will make up for your messy room."

Lisa is hardly the only person who gets turned on by a tub or other body of water. Tropical beaches, swimming pools, hot tubs, lakes, oceans, mountainside creeks, and waterfalls are all incredibly sexy locations for passion. And though they have become less popular in recent history, waterbeds have also long been a staple of sexual fantasy.

WET 'N WILD

If talking makes you feel shy, try writing! You and your partner can each make a list of things you find sexy. Swap lists and put a check mark next to the things you are comfortable exploring.

WET 'N WILD

If water turns you on, invest in a fountain or fish tank for your bedroom. Creating the perfect atmosphere sets the mood and caters to a rich fantasy life.

One of the most challenging things about connecting with a lover is discovering his or her hot spots. People can be coy, shy, or downright uncommunicative about the things that really get them going. If your sweetheart is being reticent about revealing her deepest desire or his hottest fantasy, the best thing to do is simply to ask! Though this can seem daunting (What if you hear something you aren't comfortable with? What if your partner refuses to answer your question? What if you just aren't used to talking about sex in the first place?), talking about sex is the best way to have a fulfilling sexual experience. Asking, "Baby, how can I get you hot?" or "What can I do to turn you on?" are easy ways to expand your sexual horizons. Chances are, as long as you present your query in a nonthreatening manner, a lover will be receptive to your honesty and openness.

Female Ejaculation

Female ejaculation is one of the wettest ways for a woman (and her partner) to experience sex. Unfortunately, ejaculation in women is often misunderstood, and some women who experience it fear that they are losing control of their bladders during sex play. This can be extremely embarrassing and disconcerting. But for people who love wet sex, ejaculation is a highly erotic experience. Female ejaculation occurs when a woman spurts a clear fluid from her urethra. This tends to happen during intense sexual excitement or during orgasm. This fluid is similar to the fluid produced by the prostate gland in men. It is not urine.

Though some women ejaculate during vaginal sex, for many others the contact has to be more localized in order for them to do so. For many women this means pressure has to be applied, either with a toy or a finger, directly on the G-spot. But finding that spot isn't always as easy as inserting part A into slot B and waiting for results.

The G-spot is located along the upper front wall of the vagina, about two inches in, toward the stomach. The best way to find it is by using a finger and making a "come here" motion. Women find their G-spots in different ways. Trying a variety of positions can help.

Here's a good one:

· Lie on your back with your knees bent.
· Place your feet on a bed or chair in front of you and insert a finger into your vagina. Feel the front wall of the vagina, behind the pubic bone.

· About two inches up you can find an area that feels different from the rest of surrounding skin. This area might be slightly raised, bumpy, or it might feel like a smooth walnut.
· Using your "come here" motion, gently push into the middle of this area until you find a spot that allows your finger to sink in more deeply. Because it is located on the back side of the vaginal wall, more pressure is generally needed to achieve a response.
· The area may be about the size of a pencil eraser, but it can engorge when sexually aroused to the size of a chestnut.
· Many women confuse the sensation of G-spot stimulation with the need to urinate. Try to work past this feeling and continue stimulating the area.
· For many women, doing so can result in an ejaculatory explosion.

For a sexy and educational video on the subject, check out Dr. Carol Queen's *G Marks the Spot.* Covering everything from solo exploration to the use of toys and finding the G-spot with a partner, this video is great for G-spot enthusiasts and novices alike.

Technical Details

Until the 1960s, sexuality was not considered something worthy of scientific study. That all changed when innovative sex researchers William Masters and Virginia Johnson put human subjects in a laboratory setting and monitored their journey through sexual arousal. Here's what they witnessed:

In the **arousal phase,** the heartbeat quickens and blood pressure rises. Due to increased blood flowing to the genitals, a woman's clitoris swells, and as arousal increases the vagina begins to lubricate. Often called "getting wet," this aspect of sexual arousal is key for both partners' comfort and enjoyment during sex. Men, too, experience increased blood flow to the genitals, which causes the penis to stiffen and become erect.

The body can return to an unaroused state at any time, but if sexual contact continues, the **plateau phase** begins. Contact can be focused on the genitals, but kissing, fondling, and touching any erogenous zone can maintain sexual excitement.

If arousal is maintained, climax can occur during the **orgasm phase.** The amount of arousal that is required to reach orgasm is different for everyone, but climax can be reached through almost any form of sexual stimulation, including masturbation, vaginal, oral, or anal intercourse.

After orgasm, the body returns to its normal, unaroused state. The heart rate levels out and blood pressure lowers. This is known as the **resolution phase.** As blood flow to the genital area decreases, the clitoris shrinks and penis becomes soft again.

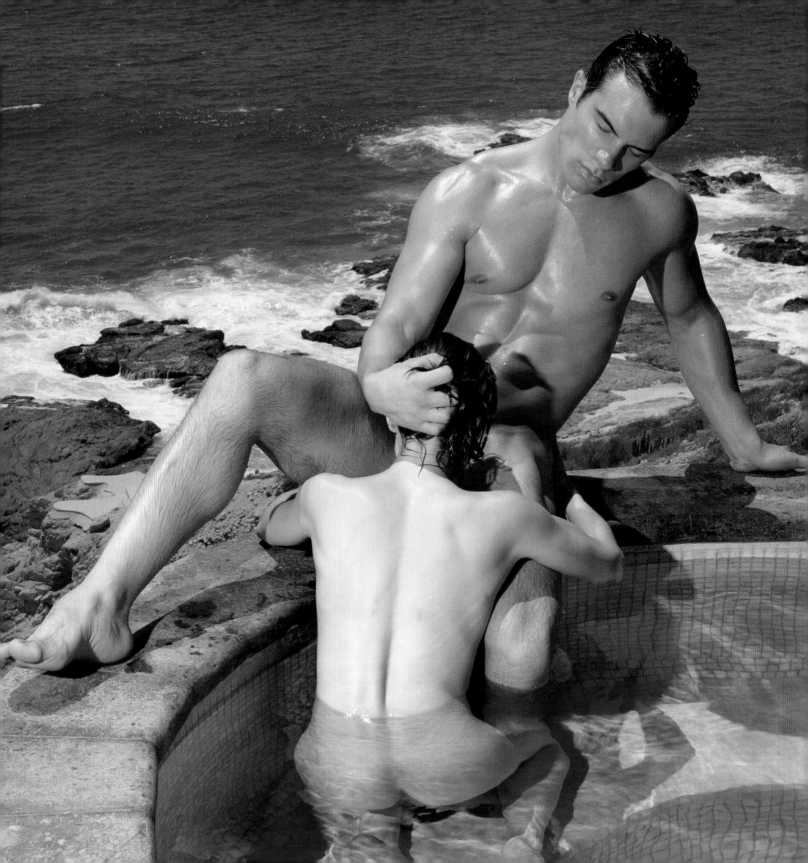

WET 'N WILD

If you are having difficulty finding the G-spot vaginally, you might be a backdoor gal. The G-spot can be indirectly stimulated through anal penetration because the vagina and the rectum are separated by only a thin membrane. Try pushing a finger, toy, or penis toward the front wall of the vagina during anal play to see if this helps you achieve G-spot stimulation.

Bridget Ejaculates

"The first time I ejaculated, I had no idea what had happened. I was kneeling facing my boyfriend who was using his hands on me. He wasn't focusing on my clitoris like he usually did, but had actually slid four fingers deep inside me. I started feeling an intense rush, not like any orgasm I had felt before. In a few seconds I felt a release, and all of a sudden water seemed to be gushing out of me. It splashed over my legs and onto the bed. It felt incredible, but I had no idea what happened. My initial reaction was to be embarrassed, but my boyfriend started rubbing the liquid all over my thighs and began kissing me and sliding his body over the wetness on mine. Then he pushed himself inside me, and we had some of the hottest sex we'd ever had. Pretty soon we figured out I had ejaculated. I loved the sensation, and he loved how wet it made sex. One of the best parts about it was that usually when I had an orgasm, I wouldn't be able to come again for a while, but if I ejaculated, I was still able to come when my clitoris was touched right afterward."

Helping Her Climax

MANY WOMEN experience frustration in trying to reach orgasm with a partner, and some women can't climax under any situation. Usually the causes are not physiological, but rather are due to inhibitions or a lack of appropriate physical stimulation. Keep these key things in mind:

• Many women do not orgasm from vaginal sex (or penetration) alone.

• Though almost any type of contact can lead to orgasm, for most women clitoral stimulation is necessary.

• For some women direct contact with the clitoris can be uncomfortable. In this case, try rubbing the vulva or lips above and around the clitoris or hold the inner lips together and slide them up and down over the clit.

• Often contact has to be direct and prolonged. Though some women can come in a matter of minutes, others will need an hour or more of direct contact in order to come.

• Hands and mouths get tired. Toys don't. Try a vibrator. The Hitachi Magic Wand has helped many women experience their first orgasm.

• Tell your partner what feels good. Lovers are not mind readers, and it is important to clearly state what you need. Saying, "I need you to go down on me before we have sex if I'm going to come," is going to get better results than simply hoping your lover figures it out.

• It can also be really helpful to show your lover what feels good and how you make yourself come.

• If you aren't getting turned on, fantasizing can help heat things up.

• Though some women love G-spot stimulation, far too many women, and their partners, focus on this area to the exclusion of the clitoris.

WET 'N WILD

Most people who have had orgasms with a partner have also made themselves come on their own. Masturbating is perfectly healthy and safe and is one of the best ways to learn what you find sexually pleasing. Once you can achieve orgasm on your own, you can more easily show a partner how to please you.

The PC Muscle

The pubococcygeus or PC muscle is a part of the body that plays a large role in sexual arousal and functioning for both men and women. The best way to find your PC muscle is to try to stop the flow of urine when using the bathroom. Once you have located the correct muscle, you can begin exercises called kegels. Kegels simply involve squeezing and releasing the PC muscle in a series of repetitions. As you progress, you will find that you are able to hold the squeeze for longer and longer. A well-developed PC muscle can intensify orgasm (when there is more muscle to tense, there is more to release), strengthen a woman's vagina, and not only help a man control the timing of his climax, but make him shoot farther when he does!

The Prostate

Women are not the only sex to lay claim to an orgasm-enhancing area. Men also possess a part of the body known for its ability to heighten sexual arousal when stimulated. This is the prostate. Though all men have this gland, not all men will enjoy having it stimulated. Unfortunately many men, who might actually enjoy the prostate, are uncomfortable with how stimulation is achieved—namely through the anus. Getting over this hang-up can do wonders for a man's sex life and can open him up to new worlds of pleasure and sensation.

Below are some tips for enhancing prostate pleasure:

· Start with a shower so you and your lover will feel clean and sensual.

· Don't immediately begin by inserting something into your man's anus. Try some other forms of foreplay first. Soap up your lover in the shower. Kiss. Cuddle. Get him hot with your hand or mouth.

· Make sure to use plenty of artificial lubricant. Unlike the vagina, the anus does not produce sufficient lube for sex play, and as always, wetter is most definitely better. Lubes like Maxxim and Anal Eze are good bets in this department.

· To locate the prostate gland, insert your finger into the anus. Push toward the front wall of the anus using the same "come here" motion discussed in G-spot play.

· In this position, the prostate can be felt through the rectal wall.

· Slowly apply pressure and see how your lover responds. Ask him if he would like you to increase pressure.

· Experiment. Find out whether he likes firm continuous pressure, or an in-and-out motion.

· Some men may enjoy prostate stimulation by itself. Others will enjoy oral sex or a handjob at the same time.

For many men, prostate massage can heighten orgasm to mind-blowing proportions. *Bend Over Boyfriend* is a sexy and educational film on the subject. For fewer lessons, but still plenty of hot sex, *Babes Ballin' Boys* might be your thing.

Cleaning Up before Getting Down 'n Dirty

Most folks know sexuality is about a whole lot more than simply thrusting for five minutes, rolling over, and then falling asleep. And getting wet is one of the best ways to mix things up. In fact, one of the sexiest preludes to sex can be a shower. Most people are not lucky enough to be in possession of the double-headed variety, but even the most cramped of shower stalls can make for a steamy clean session.

Many couples love to hold each other close as water rushes down over their sopping-wet bodies. As Matt, 30, recalls, "I think a lot of people assume that you take a shower before sex to get clean. I don't care about washing; mainly I find it sexy to shower with Allison because I love watching the water stream over her breasts and the way her hair hangs down her back when it's wet. When we get out, I'm so turned on—all I want to do is throw her on the bed."

And for people like Cathy, being washed by a lover is the most exciting part of the shower experience. "Alex loves to lather me up when we shower. He'll take a bottle of liquid soap and squeeze it all over me. Feeling his hands slide over me makes me melt. If I weren't so busy thinking about the rolling around we were going to do once we got out, I'd probably stay in the shower with him until the water went cold." Though many couples enjoy sex in the shower, for plenty of others it is the perfect warm up to a session in bed.

WET 'N WILD

If you own a waterbed, strip off the linens, replace with a plastic sheet, and slather the mattress in baby oil. The slippery sensations and rolling waves of the bed will make for a ride that is worth the mess!

Massage

Massage is always another great way to turn up the heat before getting down and dirty. Relaxing and sensual, the slickness of a partner's hands gliding across your back, over your buttocks, and down your legs can be highly arousing. Not only is massage therapeutic, but it can also be an intense turn-on for both the person applying the oil and the one receiving it. Many people become aroused just seeing their own fingers glide across a partner's skin or feeling it sink beneath their touch. For some couples a massage alone is sufficient. For others it serves as foreplay for the sex that is going to come.

Before commencing the sexiest massage imaginable, be prepared and figure out what you need. Massage oil, a towel, and moist wipes can be handy. So can candles and mood music. Make sure your hands are clean and your nails are trimmed—nothing takes you out of the mood faster than being scratched or cut! Warm up the lotion in your hands before applying it to skin; otherwise, the recipient of your soothing massage might be in for a chilly surprise.

Massage is one of the best ways to get to know a partner's entire body, not just the usual spots you encounter during sex and foreplay. Oiling up more than just your hands will make the experience that much more sensual. Using your arms, chest, and stomach as massage tools can be a great way to enhance intimacy, as well as the physical stimulation of the massage. Focusing on a lover's inner thighs, buttocks, and—if she's female—breasts, can make a massage a natural lead-up to sex play. Keep in mind that most massage oils are not designed to be used internally, so stick to lubes for any penetrative sex.

Don't rush for the towel or moist wipes before turning from massage to hot sex. Experiment with the slick skin-on-skin sensation. Often we are too quick to sanitize our sex lives, but keeping things a little down and dirty is a great way to shed inhibitions.

Scrub-a-Dub Rub

The feeling of a lover's hands gliding effortlessly across one's skin is one of the most exciting sensations ever. Skillfully using your hands to stroke and rub, tickle and tease is a surefire way to turn someone on. Hands can be divine as a pre-sex warmup, or they can be considered the main event themselves!

Getting Wet with a Woman

Many women love to have their breasts caressed, and both men and women can be brought to heightened states of ecstasy by having their nipples teased and taunted. Hands can travel down to a backside for a squeeze and then slide forward to caress a lover's nether regions. When touching the genitals, most people prefer a slippery sensation. Generally, the vagina produces lubrication when a woman becomes sexually aroused. However, some women may not become wet enough to enjoy being touched or entered. Medications, hormonal birth control, age, and a lack of foreplay can all contribute to this situation. But don't despair. Break out an artificial lubricant. Lubes stay wet even when you don't. They can make penetration more comfortable, reduce unpleasant friction, and heighten sensation. Dribbling a lubricant between a lover's legs is a highly erotic act, and many women adore the feeling of fingers trailing smoothly across their clitoris or slowly sliding over their labia before entering them. These tips will help you caress your lady the right way:

· If your partner isn't wet, make sure to get her there with some artificial lube.

· The clitoris is the most concentrated site of nerve endings in the genitals. Some women love firm pressure on their clitoris. For others, a more gentle or indirect touch is needed.

· As you touch her clitoris, ask her how it feels.

· If she likes a direct touch, you can rub her in a circular or up-and-down motion.

· If she prefers less contact, try rubbing her clitoris through her inner labia or with the wider heel of your hand.

· Though guys often want the rhythm to speed up before they climax, for many women the motion has to be steady. Changing pace can disrupt a gal's flow and keep her orgasm at bay.

· A lot of women like a finger (or two or three) inserted into their vagina while the clitoris is being stimulated. Some woman simply like the pressure this adds. Others crave strong thrusting.

· Ditto for the anus.

· If things don't seem as slippery as they had been a moment before, add more lube as you go. Different brands will stay wet for longer or shorter periods. If there is too much, simply wipe away excess with a towel or moist wipe.

· There's no reason not to make her come with your hand even if you are planning on more sex play. Unlike men, women can have numerous orgasms in a short period of time!

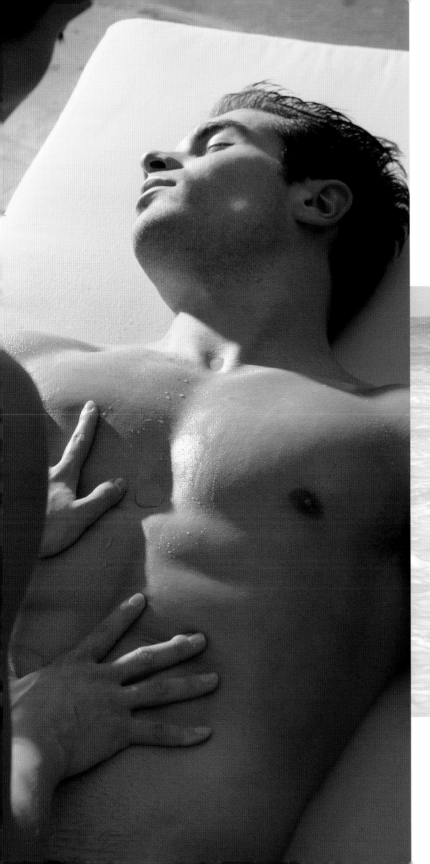

Aquatic Massage

An aquatic massage is a liquid take on traditional massage therapy. Allowing yourself to sink into an aquatic massage can expand your understanding of your body while providing a gentle, hands-on experience that takes advantage of the anti-gravity properties of water. The body experiences a larger range of motion in the water than it does on dry land. During an aquatic massage, you float on your back while the water helps the masseuse support you. Individuals often experience an increased appreciation both of the powers of water as well as of their own bodies when they are experiencing the warm, gentle freedom of motion that aquatic massage permits. During a Watsu style aquatic massage, gentle Shiatsu stretches increase flexibility while you float in the calm warm water. The massage involves a focus on deep breathing and is often called "water breath dance" in reference to the movements your body will make through the water.

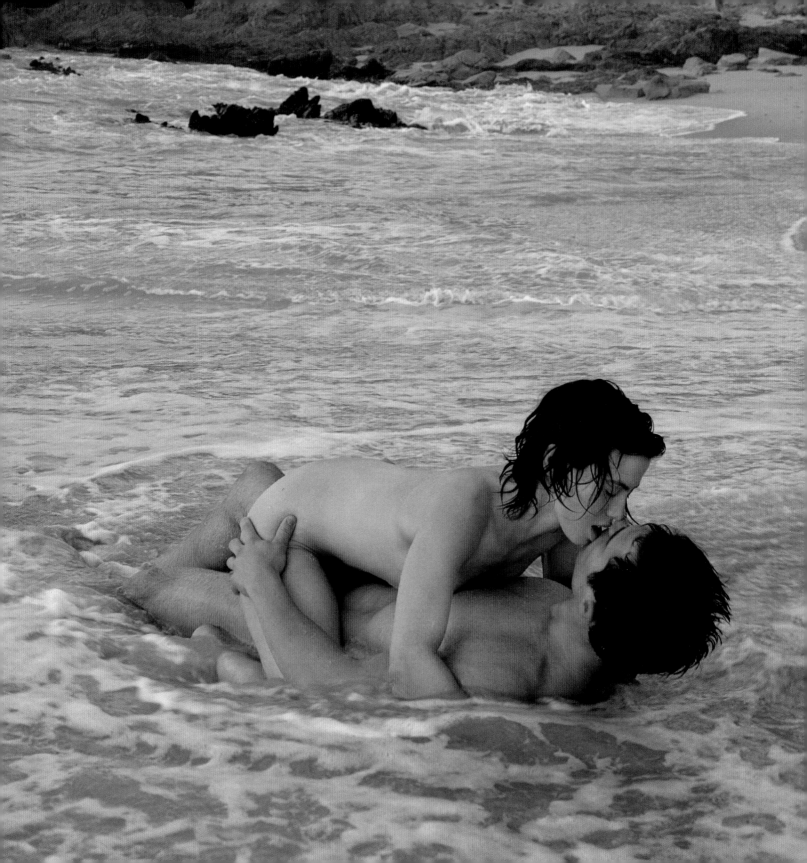

Getting Wet with a Man

Lube is also key when giving handjobs. Unlike the vagina, the penis does not produce natural lubrication besides a negligible amount of pre-cum. Nevertheless, most guys agree that any hand contact is greatly enhanced by a smooth, gliding sensation. As Paul, 38, relates, "Sometimes women don't realize how uncomfortable it is to get jacked-off dry. When her hand slips over me it feels amazing, but rubbing up and down without lube makes me feel raw and sore." Sometimes people are shy about using lubricants, but doing so is one the easiest (and wettest) ways to enhance pleasure.

It's easy to forget how hot a handjob can be. Many men's first experiences with handjobs were fumbling teenage affairs that lacked the benefit of lube, or know how. But when done properly, a handjob is a sexy act for people of all ages. Handjobs let you look into your partner's eyes. They provide the perfect position for deep kissing and whispering into a lover's ears. Whether you are trying to get him hot or get him off, hands are far sexier than they are often given credit for. Here are some handjob helpers:

· Don't worry if he isn't rock hard when you start. Often the touch of your hand will be all he needs. If he still isn't hard, take the focus off his penis for a few minutes. Kiss and caress. Let him feel your breasts against him and nibble on his neck or ear to help get things going.

· Once he's hard, get him wet. Saliva works for this. So does artificial lube. A lot of guys use moisturizer or Vaseline when they masturbate. These are fine for handjobs as long as you aren't using a latex condom (which can break when it comes into contact with an oil-based product).

· There are many different ways to grip a man's penis. Many people start by holding the penis and sliding their hand up and down the shaft.

· If a man has foreskin, ask if his head is too sensitive for direct touch. If he says yes, make sure the foreskin covers the glans as you stroke him. If he says no, he might prefer his foreskin rolled back during sex play.

· The head of the penis is the most sensitive part of the organ. Lingering at the head on the upstroke and running your thumb around the frenulum (the ridged area that separates a guy's head from his shaft) is often very pleasurable.

· Women are often surprised at how firmly men grip their penises and how rapidly they stroke themselves. Ask your guy if he wants increased pressure or speed.

· If he dries up, add more lube!

· A lot of guys enjoy the feeling of a finger in their anus during handjobs. Ask first and use a lot of lube. In you have long fingernails, you might want to hold off on this one. That is definitely not the place for an accidental cut.

· Ask him whether there is someplace special where he wants to come and continue stroking him to an earth-shattering climax.

Waterproof Lubricants

Sex in the water is one of the hottest experiences around. Unfortunately, water can also wash away a woman's natural vaginal lubrication and make for some pretty raw sensations. Luckily, silicone-based lubricants stay wet even when you're not. Unlike water-based lubes, which will just wash away, silicone lubricants are perfect for use in hot tubs, pools, the ocean, or even in the bath. Brands like Eros Bodyglide and Pink Lube are perfect for comfortable, underwater sex. A petroleum-based lubricant, like Wet's mineral oil and Vitamin E variety, though not as good for underwater adventures, can be used in a shower or when your aren't planning on a fully saturated experience. Remember, never use an oil-based lube with a latex condom!

Getting Wet with Oral Sex

Hot, wet, and sexy, the mouth is an amazing part of our anatomy. The vision of moist, slightly parted lips opening to receive a drinking straw, a chocolate-covered cherry, or even a cigarette can be all it takes to drive your lover wild. The mouth is sensual without even trying. But when it tries, oh does it deliver! Oral sex, once a taboo known as the "French Perversion" is now a staple of many people's sexual encounters. Using your mouth to stimulate a lover's genitals is a slippery, slick ride and one of the most intimate sex acts a couple can engage in. It is also fairly easy to incorporate into many different settings. Bathtubs, pools, and the beach can all lend themselves discrete (or not so discrete) blowjobs and labial licks.

Whether you choose to lie back and relax as your lover's lips and tongue pleasure you or spin around for some sixty-nine action, oral sex can get you ready for the next course, or bring you to orgasm right then and there.

Mellie, 26, says, "I love it when my boyfriend goes down on me. I get really excited by the idea, so when it actually happens I go crazy. When I pull him up to kiss me, he knows that's a signal that I'm ready to screw."

Greg, 41, only began enjoying blowjobs as he got older. "I was really inhibited with my wife. We got married right after college and had never slept with anyone else. She went down on me a few times, but she didn't seem to like it, so I never pushed the issue. After we spilt up and I started dating, I found out what I had been missing! I kind of feel like I am making up for lost time now. I'd almost be as happy with head as I would be with sex."

For some people, the sexiness of a blowjob is partly visual. "I love pornos where girls can get a stringer of saliva from their mouth to the guy's dick," says Lainey, 22. "It looks so sloppy and wet and like they just want to get him off and make a mess."

The attraction of the visual element is very common. As Brandon, 33, explains, "I never want to come in a girl's mouth. Both my girlfriend and I like to watch myself come, which makes our orgasms even more intense."

When we think about what it entails, it's no surprise that oral sex is so appealing. The combination of a wet mouth on wet genitals—producing amazing orgasmic sensations—just can't be beat.

WET 'N WILD

One thing that can kill oral sex is the dreaded dry mouth. This is often brought on by nerves, dehydration, or booze. Keep a glass of water on hand for an instant fix.

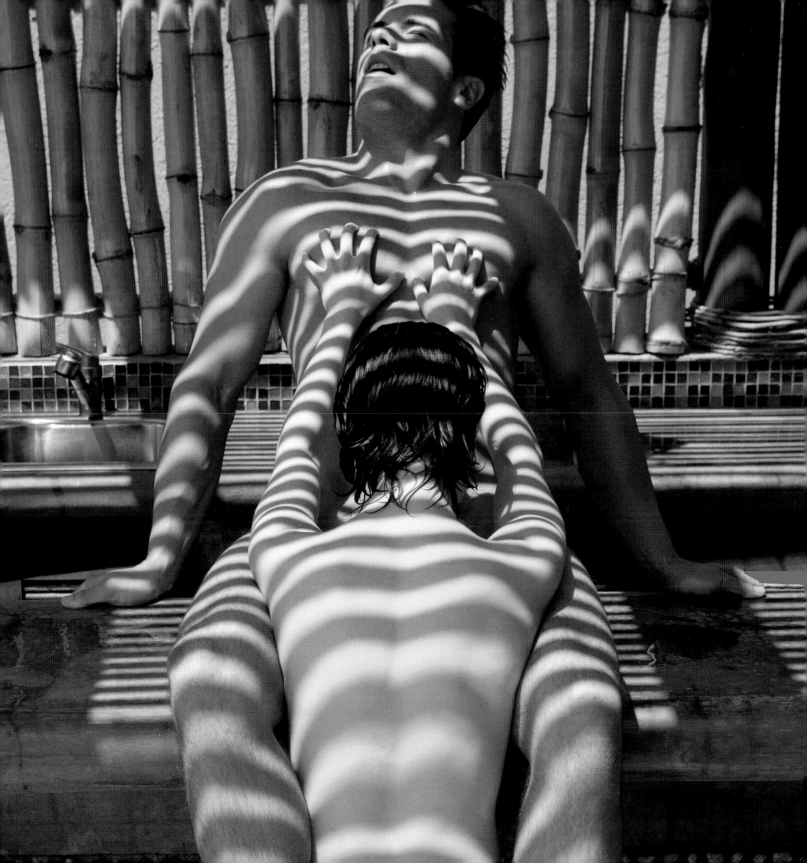

Oral Sex for Beginners

There you are, head between a lover's legs, but instead of diving in, all you can think is, "What do I do now?" There's no doubt: Oral sex can be intimidating. People often fear that their mouth won't be sufficient to make a lover moan. In reality, licking a lover, like any other sex act, is best enhanced by a little skill and a lot of communication.

Going Down on Gals

Every woman has a different way she likes to be touched, but having her vagina caressed by a lover's tongue is something most women delight in. Try these ideas for going down on the gals:

· With a wet tongue, trace her labia and glide your way up to her clitoris.

· Using your tongue to lick and your lips to suck, work this organ while stroking her inner thighs and lips.

· Some gals enjoy a finger or toy inside them while you're using your mouth; for others this will be a distraction. Find out what your lady prefers by asking.

· When it comes to oral sex, the ability to take direction is key.

· Don't be offended if she asks you to go slower or faster, to use more tongue, less teeth, or a circular motion. Each woman's body responds to different types of touch, and there is no way to know which strokes will work best for a particular person without some hints.

WET 'N WILD

If you always do it in the dark, try illuminating the situation by keeping the lights on. Remember that your body drenched in sweat is an utterly delicious sight for your lover's eyes, no matter how shy about it you might feel.

Going Down on Guys

Like going down on a woman, going down on a man can be a little nerve wracking. Women often worry about gagging, biting, or otherwise making a mess of things. But making a mess isn't always bad. Sloppy, slobbery head can be sexy and fun! Here are some helpful hints:

· Don't start by forcing his entire penis into your mouth.

· Begin by licking your partner's scrotum and shaft. This can get him nice and slick. It can also increase anticipation and heighten sensitivity.

· Though some guys go crazy for deep-throat action, most men are perfectly content if you take into your mouth what fits comfortably.

· From the front of the mouth to the back of the throat is about five inches or so. The average erect penis is about five to seven inches. If his penis is too long for your mouth, don't despair! That's what hands are for. Use your hand to hold the remainder of his shaft. If you make sure your hand and mouth are working in tandem to slide up and down his penis, it is unlikely you will hear any complaints.

· Use your tongue to lick and tease the head of his penis and run it around the frenulum.

Some guys like to come in their partner's mouth and see their lover swallow their load, but not everyone is comfortable with this. If you're not, you can always spit out the semen or avoid taking it into your mouth in the first place. Remember, plenty of guys get off on watching their cum shoot out onto other areas. Another option is to have a man wear a condom. This is a great way to avoid taking ejaculate into the mouth and is also a good safety precaution.

Off the Beaten Track

MANY PEOPLE ARE SEXUALLY AROUSED by niche fantasies and sexual practices, which are often called fetishes or paraphilias. These terms refer to sexual arousal that occurs in response to objects, situations, or forms of nonmainstream sexual expression. Though individuals with fetishes have long been viewed with suspicion, most fetishists do not harm others. Almost anything can be eroticized, and water is no exception. Fetishes that involve wetness include:

Water Sports

The term "water sports" refers to a sex practice called urophilia. More commonly known as "golden showers," this type of sex play generally involves one partner urinating in front of or on the other. The appeal of water sports is varied. For some people, water sports break deep-seated taboos, for others the enjoyment lies in the complete abandonment of worries about hygiene. Some researchers even believe that urine itself can actually be an aphrodisiac!

Wet Panties

Wet panty enthusiasts are aroused by someone wearing wet underwear. Whether dampened by urine or sexual fluids, the Internet lists scores of sites devoted to wet panties. People are taught from an early age not to wet their pants, and that doing so is not only wrong and naughty, but unhygienic and embarrassing. Wet panty enthusiasts turn these notions on their heads to make sexy what others find distasteful.

Sploshing

Sploshing is all about getting wet and dirty. Sometimes called messy sex, or wamming (from wet and messy), sploshing enthusiasts roll around and cover themselves in food, mud, shaving cream, and other substances. Sometimes sploshers have sex while coated in substances, but often the enjoyment is found in the sploshing itself without the addition of sex play.

Wetlook

Fans of wetlook find people wearing soaking wet clothes incredibly arousing. Erotic videos catering to this theme feature women submerged in swimming pools while wearing business suits, as well as a more classic vision: the drenched girl in a wet t-shirt.

Water Bondage

Water bondage is a variation of dry-land bondage. During water bondage, participants are either tied up underwater and given scuba gear to breathe, or they are bound in a more traditional setting and then are hosed down with water. Some water bondage involves bringing someone to a "water orgasm." This means using a stream of water on an immobilized person's genitals until climax occurs.

Mud Wrestling

Wrestling has long been a popular sport, and although many in the professional wrestling world would deny it, much of the appeal lies in watching two people grappling with each other until one becomes the victor. Adding a slippery element like mud and a skimpy bathing suit can make a wrestling session all the more hot, both for the participants and the observers.

The Scoop on Fluids

The body is an amazing thing. Though you would never know it from looking at someone, much of what we are is actually liquid. This is because the majority of our body is composed of water. We also produce various other fluids during sex play, including vaginal secretions, semen, and sweat. Of course, how these fluids taste and smell can affect a lover's response and your experience. But because what we put into our body has a direct effect on what comes out, the quality of your bodily fluids is not completely out of your control. To become as tasty as possible, avoid things like caffeine, alcohol, and garlic, and indulge in fruits like grapefruit, pineapple, and limes. And always remember to drink plenty of water. Water flushes out toxins in the body. A little thing like keeping hydrated will help you smell and taste delicious!

Audacia Ray, Messy Wrestler

Audacia Ray is a writer, sex-worker-rights advocate, alternative model, and safer-sex educator. She has also had plenty of experience with messy wrestling—wrestling in various wet and goopy substances. After rolling around with other women in everything from fake blood to oil to a mysterious green slime, Audacia became a bit of an expert on the subject. She says, "I think people find messy wrestling sexy for two reasons. First, wetness emphasizes the body in a really cool, really sexy way, especially if there's some clothing being worn. Also, it's sexy because of the slippery factor—wet bodies sliding over each other is pretty exciting." For more about Audacia, check out www.wakingvixen.com.

Aquatic Fun and Games

A great way to get into a sexy mood is to heat things up with some wet, hot forePLAY! Games are a great way to introduce new ideas and to liven up an erotic encounter. If you're looking to add some liquid to your lovemaking, here are a few suggestions:

Catch Me If You Can

Hop into a pool and blindfold your lover. Entice him or her to find you solely based on your calls of *hotter* and *colder*. Once you are found, reward your honey with a kiss, an underwater grope, or a naughty nibble!

Ice Is Nice

Break out the ice tray for a slippery ride across your lover's body. Ice can be run sensuously down hot thighs, over buttocks, and across taunt nipples for heightened sensation and stimulation. Try putting a cube or two in your mouth for oral sex and delight in the sensation of it melting over your lover's warm flesh. Just make sure to keep anything frozen external.

Write It Out

Use massage oil to spell out instruction on your honey's back. Try a product like Kiss of Fire Edible Warming Massage Oil to spell out instructions directing your partner to do your bidding. If your lover can't figure out what you've written, he has to perform the act! If he can, a massage is the reward.

Naughty Dice

Naughty dice, which have erotic phrases written in place of numbers, are always a fun way to get a night started. When they are rolled together, the combinations spell out instructions for lovers like, "kiss" "ear". Water lovers can make up their own naughty dice wet game by creating two lists from numbered 1 to 6.

List One:
1) *Lick*
2) *Suck*
3) *Ice*
4) *Kiss*
5) *Spray*
6) *Tickle*

List Two:
1) *Nipples*
2) *Mouth*
3) *Penis*
4) *Vulva*
5) *Buttocks*
6) *Thighs*

For example, if you roll a 5 and a 1, then you would use a spray bottle on your partner's nipples. A 3 and a 6 could find you trailing ice up his thighs, and so on. Don't forget any necessary props.

WET 'N WILD

Try waking your lover up with caresses from your tongue. Work your way down from the neck to the chest to the abdomen to the genitals for an utterly delicious start to the day!

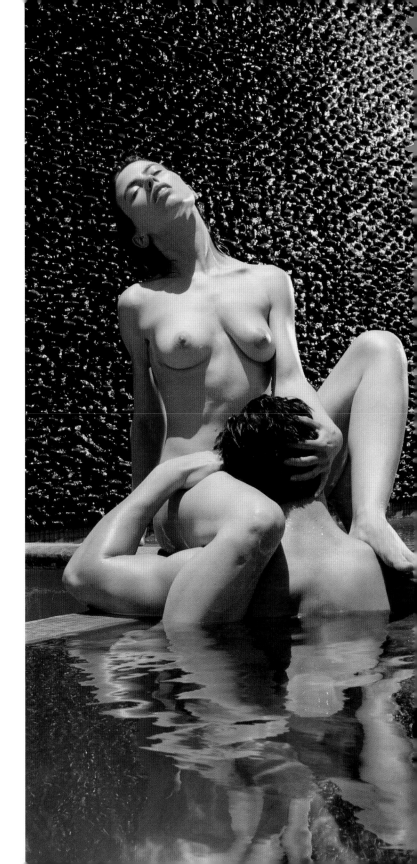

Underwater Striptease

For the more daring, challenge your partner to fully remove his or her bathing suit in a public pool or ocean and get it back on without anyone else noticing. You can cop a few underwater feels if you're quick!

Wrestle Mania

Lay down thick towels or mats. Cover these with a big plastic sheet or tarp. Coat each other in baby oil from head to toe. Then proceed to have your own personal wrestling match. Feel free to make up your own rules. You can decide that two tumbles decide a win or that shoulders have to be pinned for ten seconds in order to score a point. The loser will be required to give the winner a thorough sponge bath.

Body Paint Party

Body paint is a fun and exciting way to decorate your lover's most intimate parts. Sexy and sensual, you can use a brush or your fingers. Make sure to use paint specifically for the purposes of decoration. Then hop into the shower together for a sexy clean-up session. For a variation on paint, try liquid latex designed for body decoration.

Sexy Sandcastles

Sand can hold heat and mold itself to the contours of your body. Challenge your lover to make sexy sand imprints. Then take digital pictures of your creations for future enjoyment.

WET 'N WILD

Try dribbling chocolate sauce or honey over your lover's body for an exciting edible experience.

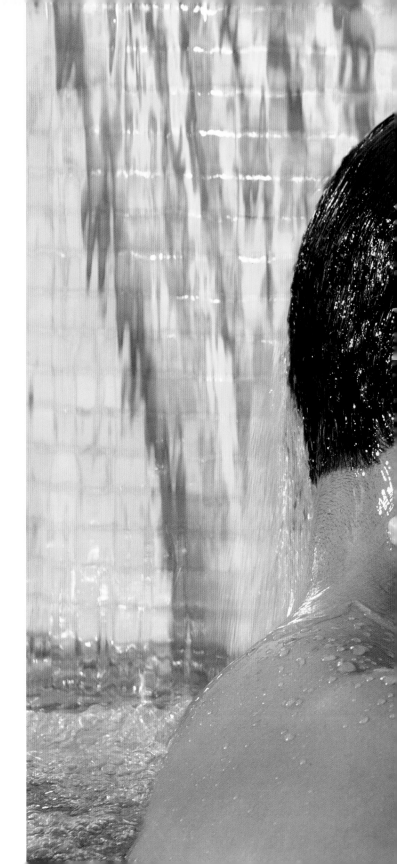

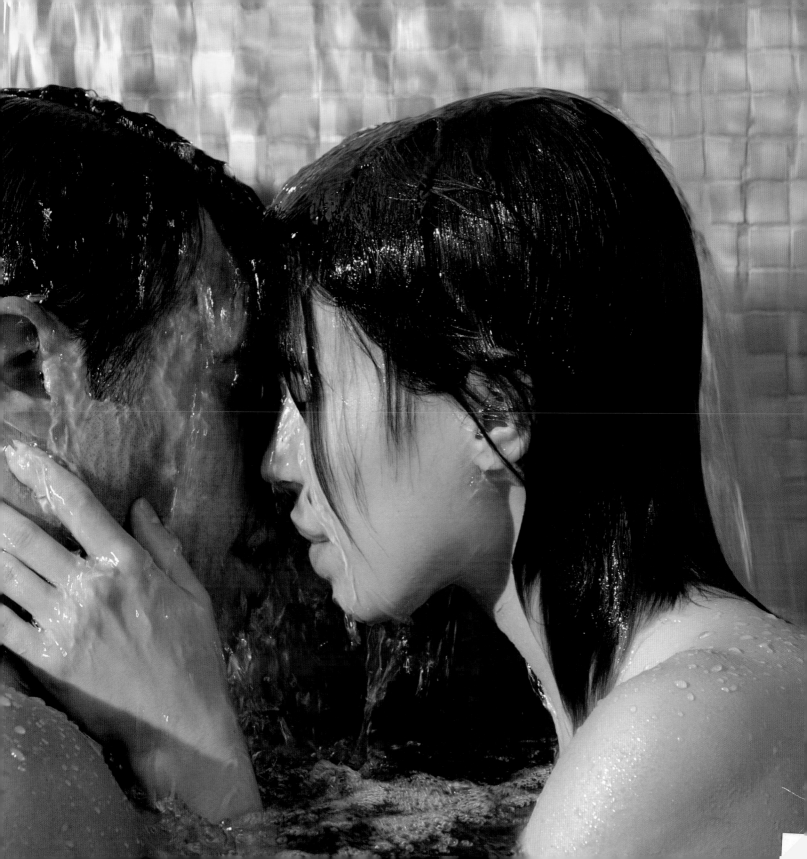

Role Playing

Poll any number of people about what they find hot, and chances are you will hear plenty of waterlogged fantasies. The connection between wetness and sex is a powerful one. Role playing is a fantastic way to mix up your usual sexual encounters and explore fantasies that would otherwise be unattainable. When you effectively step into a role, you can shed inhibitions and become a completely new person. Many people don't realize that they already play roles during their sex play. They might become more coy, aggressive, or shy than they are in other settings. However, when you consciously dive into a role-play scenario, you can overcome some of the hang-ups and overcompensations that thwart your sexual freedom and replace them with a bold, seductive new you.

Many people are embarrassed to try role playing, thinking they will feel foolish or embarrass themselves. Don't be discouraged if you or your lover let out a giggle or two. Often laughter is a product of nerves and not a sign that your idea or performance is being mocked. To start a role play, think about a scene that turns you on. It doesn't have to be elaborate, but it should be something that excites you and your lover.

Here are some aqueous role-playing ideas you might find exciting:

Pirate/Captive Maiden

Though they are helpful, you don't need an eye patch or hook for a hand to step into this role. Simply set the stage by threatening to tie up your captive, or tell her she'll have to walk the plank unless she succumbs to your desires.

Sailor Out on the Town

Plenty of people love a man in uniform. Buy or rent a sailor suit and pretend you have just picked up your lover at a seedy bar. Prepare for a wild night of sex with a stranger before you set sail for ports unknown in the morning.

Don't I Know You from Somewhere?

Agree to meet at your favorite beach and act as if you don't know each other. Flirt with your honey shamelessly. Use fake names if it will help get you in the mood. Then find a secluded spot for hot sex. Have a quickie and leave separately. You might have been together for ten years, but sex under these circumstances will make it seem like the first time.

Nurse, It's Time for My Sponge Bath . . .

Get your sweetie to dress up in a hot little nurse's outfit. The shorter and more revealing the better! Have her run a bath for you. She can be naughty or nice, stern or sweet, but either way, a thorough nurse knows that all a patient's parts need to be squeaky clean before he is allowed to leave the tub. Inspections might be necessary and rewards for good behavior can be offered.

Though it can take a little getting used to, slipping into a different role will come more naturally if you let your inhibitions down and remind yourself that sex doesn't always have to be serious. Remember, you aren't auditioning for a major Hollywood film, you are simply enjoying sex play with a lover.

"*A girlfriend* gave me a set of *edible body paints* as a joke for my bachelorette party. One night I was feeling a little frisky, and I pulled them out and started painting different body parts of my husband while he read his book. Well, once I started *touching those sensitive areas*—his nipples, *his chest,* and his penis—he became very excited. Needless to say, he dropped his book as I started to *lick the paint off!*"

—Alison, 32

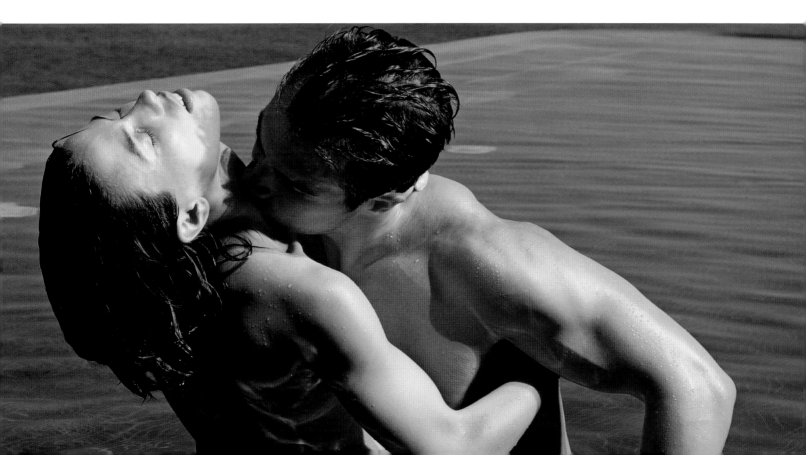

WET 'N WILD

Make your lover an aquatically
arousing gift basket. Include a
waterproof vibrator, a spray
bottle, a sponge, an erotic
bathtub read, lubricants, a
bottle of champagne, and
anything else that you think
will be a good addition to
sexy, wet fun.

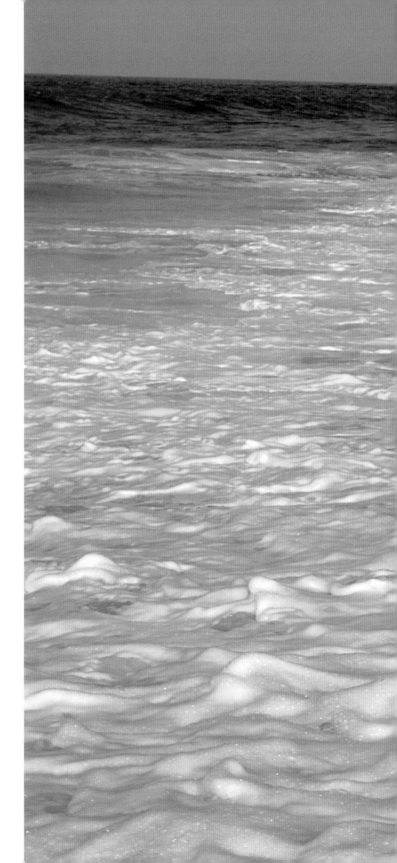

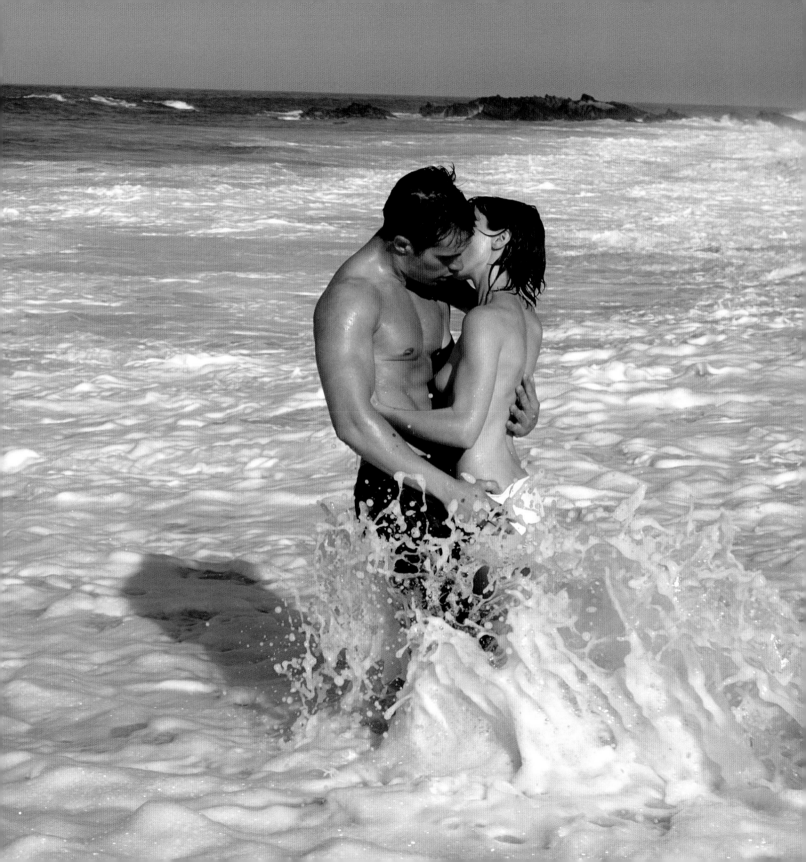

Toys

If you think toys are just for kids, think again! There are plenty of adult toys just waiting to be played with. So if water is your thing, then you're in luck, as many of these toys are actually waterproof.

But why use a sex toy in the first place? Sex toys can enhance a sexual experience. They can throw a kink into your routine, and they can allow for exploration and experimentation. Sex toys can give you the chance to switch roles with a partner, or ditch the need for a partner altogether. And while people can grow tired, a toy can last all night. But above all, sex toys are just plain fun!

Vibrators and Dildos

Two of the most common toys are vibrators and dildos. Vibrators come in different shapes and sizes; they may oscillate, throb, pulsate, or quiver; and they can be used anywhere on the body that feels good. Women often use them for clitoral stimulation, but they also can be used on nipples or inside vaginas and anuses. Many men like the sensation of vibration on their penis, perineum, anus, or scrotum. Dildos, on the other hand, don't vibrate. Shaped like a phallus for easy penetration, a dildo can be used instead of a penis for vaginal, anal, and even oral sex.

Both vibrators and dildos can be used alone or with a partner, either by themselves or in conjunction with other forms of sex play. For example, some people love wearing a butt-plug to stimulate the anus while getting a handjob or having vaginal sex. And many women use vibrators during vaginal sex to help them climax while a partner is inside them. Long gone are the days when sex toys were thought only to be used by lonely perverts who couldn't get a date! Today we know that toys can enhance sex in myriad ways for anyone who cares to dabble.

Sharice recalls the messages she heard about sex toys growing up. "I remember walking by a sex shop with my mom as a kid. She told me anyone who shopped there was dirty. It took my boyfriend a long time to convince me that using a vibrator wouldn't make me dirty, it would just make sex better."

Sadly, far too many people grow up with the idea that sex is something to be kept under wraps and expressed in a very limited fashion. Remind yourself that as long as it is safe and consensual, it is perfectly fine to enhance your sex life as you see fit, whether it is by using a toy, tying up a lover, or have mind-blowing orgasms underwater!

Toys intensify sexual encounters and add a dash of spice to a strictly vanilla scene, but there are a few things for water lovers (and others) to keep in mind:

· Even if a toy is sold as waterproof, it might not take kindly to hot tub chemicals or pool chlorine. In a pool or hot tub, avoid using your Cyberskin dildo and stick to the less-delicate plastic toys.

· Enjoying your toy in the ocean? Make sure not to let it slip from your hand under the pressure of an oncoming wave or wake from a boat.

· Most toys work better with lube. Silicone lubes work better in the water than water-based ones, which will simply wash away.

· Test your toy out somewhere safe (like the kitchen sink) before you plunge it into the bath with you. Some toys are only "splash-proof" and should not be submerged.

· Keep your toys clean. Waterproof toys are easy to care for—just wash and dry. For a longer shelf life, remember to take the batteries out between uses as well.

· Sharing toys? Wash well between uses or, even better, cover with a condom.

· Only use toys anally that have a wide enough base to prevent them from slipping inside the body.

Water Friendly Sex Toys!

WATER ENTHUSIASTS WILL BE HAPPY TO KNOW that sex toys are not just the domain of those who prefer to do it on dry land. Almost all dildos are water friendly, as are any other plastic, glass, or acrylic toys that don't have a cord or battery. There are also plenty of battery-operated toys specifically designed for water play. In fact, www.mypleasure.com lists sixty, www.xandria.com lists fifty-nine, and www.babeland.com lists thirty-nine battery-operated toys that can be used in the water!

VIBRATORS

Love G
This waterproof vibe has 10 levels of vibration and pulsation. It's thick and angled at the tip for G-spot exploration, and it is textured throughout for heightened internal and clitoral sensations.

Men's Pleasure Wand
This vibrator, designed just for men, has a curved shape that can stimulate the scrotum and prostate at the same time.

Sea Lover
A multi-speed vibrator designed to look like a penis and testicles.

Velvet Contour
Perfect for anal play, this vibrator boasts varying speeds and is angled to increased prostate stimulation. With a flared base, it doesn't run the risk of slipping inside the body.

Passion Lily
A bullet-shaped vibrator covered in a soft sleeve in the shape of a blooming flower. Good for both vaginal and clitoral stimulation.

Finger Fun Vibrator
A vibrator that fits unobtrusively on one finger and is made of clear jelly rubber.

Water Dancer
The traditional pocket rocket vibrator made especially for water play.

DILDOS

Silicone
A premium material, silicone is easy to clean, warms quickly, and comes in an array of colors.

Acrylic, glass, and metal
These are made of the hardest stuff around! Though not lifelike in texture, they make up for in being able to deliver in power.

Cyberskin
As close to the real thing as you can get, these dildos are made of lifelike materials called cyberskin or ultraskin. Make sure to dust them off with cornstarch after use to prevent your toy from getting sticky.

OTHER

Waterproof nipple and testicle teaser
Vibrating cups that can be placed over the nipples or testicles.

Waterproof anal beads
Waterproof beads that can be inserted into the anus for stimulation. Some varieties include a waterproof vibrator in the tip.

Little Zinger butt plug
This butt plug can be inserted in or out of the water for a sensation of fullness and prostate stimulation.

Waterproof vibrating lips
These sponge-like lips are equipped with a vibrator. Good for use on her clitoris or as a warm wet home for his penis.

Vibrating cock ring
A natural buzz! This cock ring can be worn face up to stimulate her clitoris during sex, or turn it around to hit his perineum.

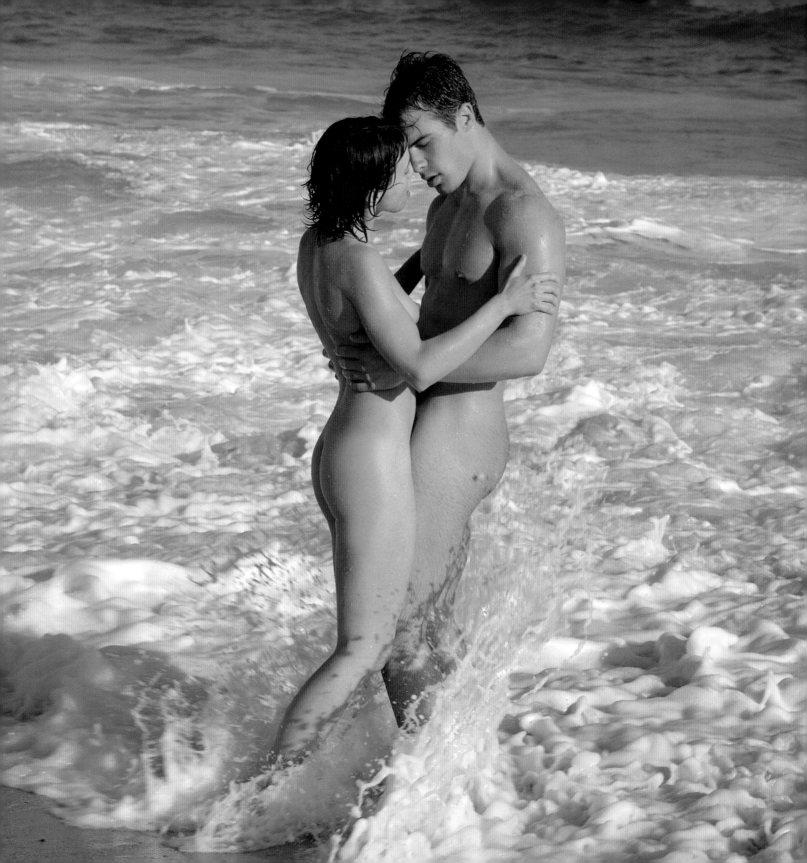

The Hidden Treasure of Underwater Orgasms

Underwater orgasms can be a new take on climaxing. The sensation of floating and feeling weightless can be just what you need to get over the edge and experience a euphoric rush. Mandy, 29, says, "I love to make myself climax in the tub. Being surrounded by water as I orgasm makes me feel so incredibly relaxed and sexy."

Eliza remembers one of her most intense orgasms happening while on vacation. "I was in Hawaii with my boyfriend. We had made it a goal to do it in the water. One night we went out to the beach. It wasn't totally deserted, but it was dark and no one seemed to notice us. We swam for a while and then we found a spot by a pier. My boyfriend leaned against it and I straddled him while he held me up. I kept my bathing suit on, but just pulled it over so he could slide into me. I don't normally come when I'm on top, but I think being submerged in this warm water made the whole situation seem sexy and safe. That was one of the most intense orgasms I've ever had."

For people who are used to having sex on a bed in the dark, introducing the element of water is a great way to shed the inhibitions that far too often hold back the pleasure we are capable of having.

Coming underwater can be more intense than coming on land for a few reasons:

· The physical awareness of water surrounding your entire body.

· Heightened sensation.

· A feeling of weightlessness.

· The mingling of your body fluids with the fluids surrounding you.

· In colder temperatures, experiencing the contrast between the warmth coursing through your body, and the chill of the water surrounding you. Everyone has different ways in which they like to climax. Even if you are completely satisfied with your dry-land orgasms, it is worthwhile to try for an underwater one. Water is an amazing conduit for sexual energy and exploration, and you might be surprised by the results of a little experimentation.

WET 'N WILD

Though you might think a toy is a great thing to have on a vacation, airport security won't always agree. To avoid hassles, embarrassment, or confiscation, pack your toys in your checked luggage. And consider removing any batteries to avoid having luggage that hums!

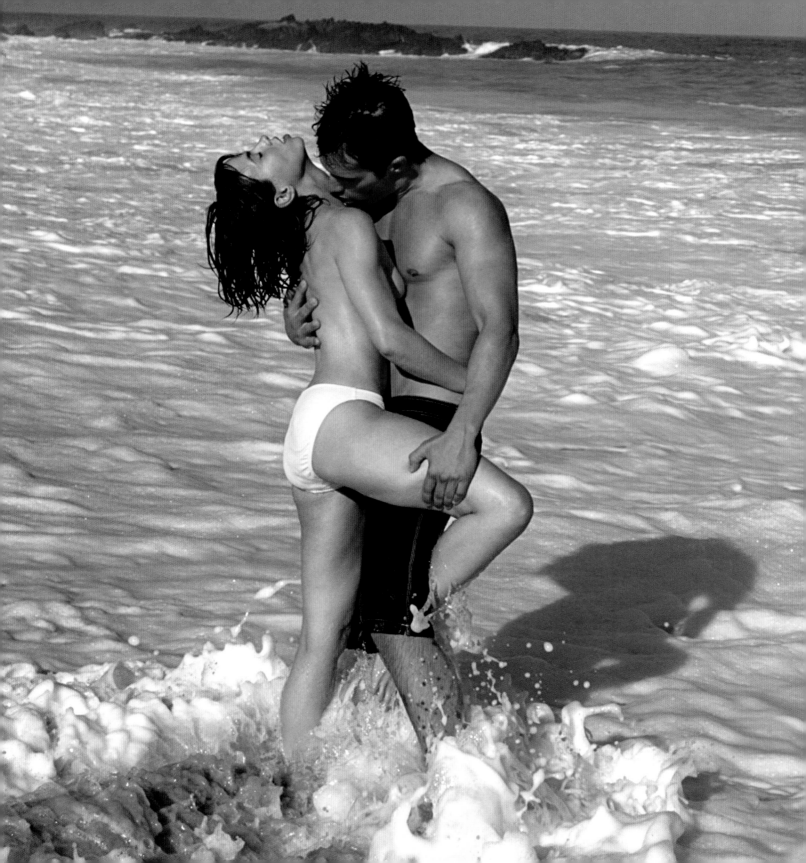

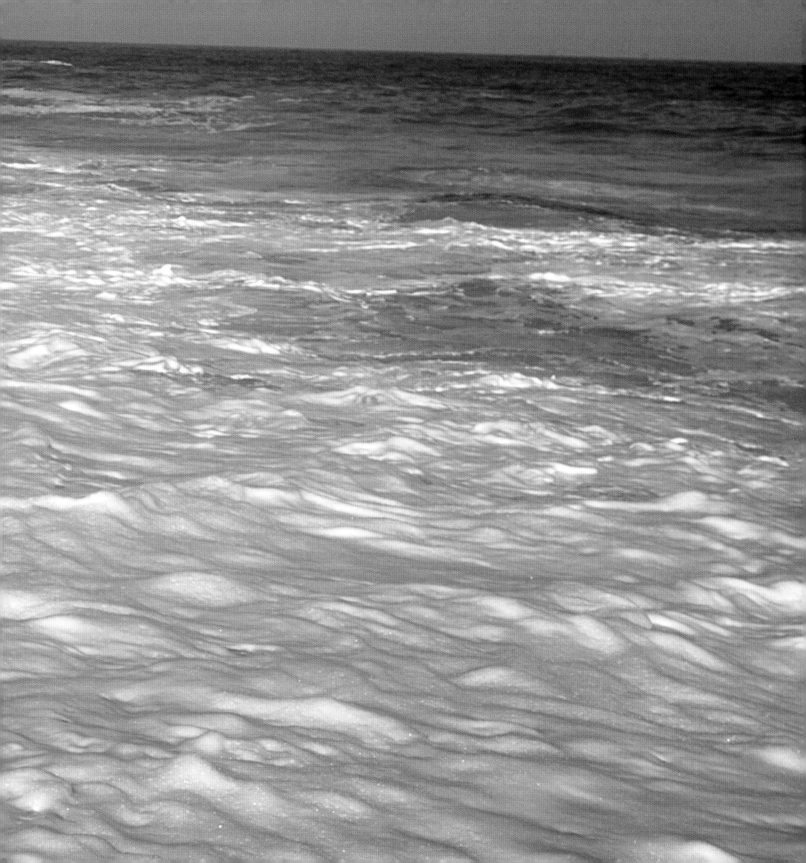

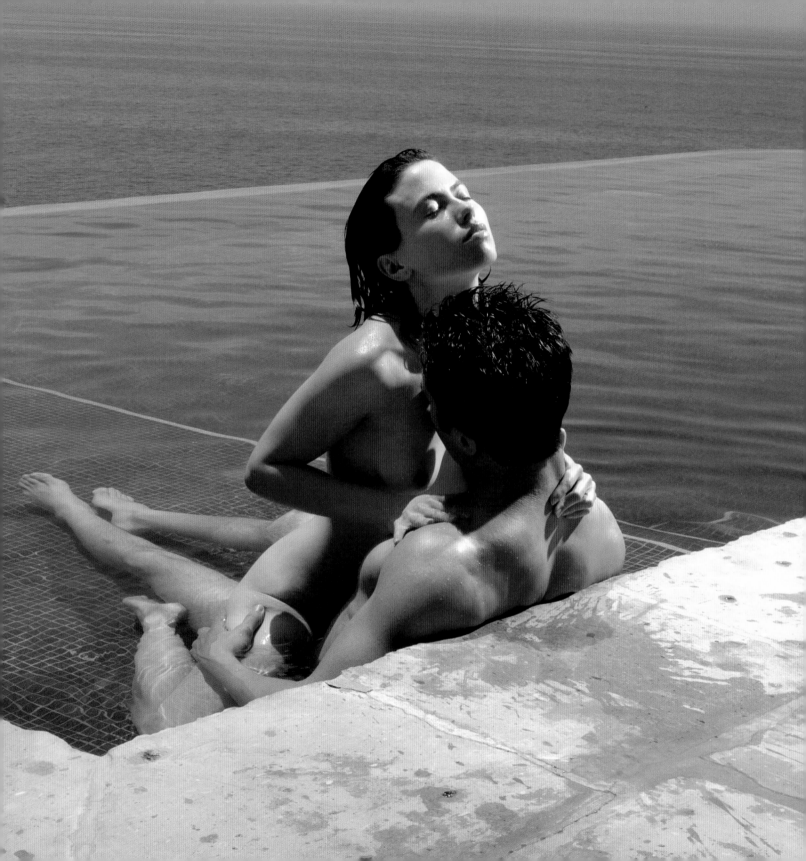

Ahhh, Arousal . . .

We live in a goal-oriented, fast-paced society, but sex is not a competition or a race. It should be savored, enjoyed, and explored. There are countless ways to heighten passion and increase pleasure. Sometimes we just need to take the time to let our imaginations run wild. Aqueous sex play allows for countless routes of exploration and adventure. Though you might be an old hand at role playing, choosing a nautical theme for your scenes can add a completely new element to your sessions. Similarly, no matter how many showers you have taken in your life, nothing can compare to showering with a lover. Mixing up your usual routine with toys, games, and even new sex acts is one of the best ways to make your sex life that much more exciting and fulfilling. With a little creativity and a lot of water, your sex life is bound to take you on a wild, wet ride.

WET 'N WILD

Practice your underwater orgasm alone in the tub. Once you have mastered your technique, invite your sweetie in to join you for a little lesson in love!

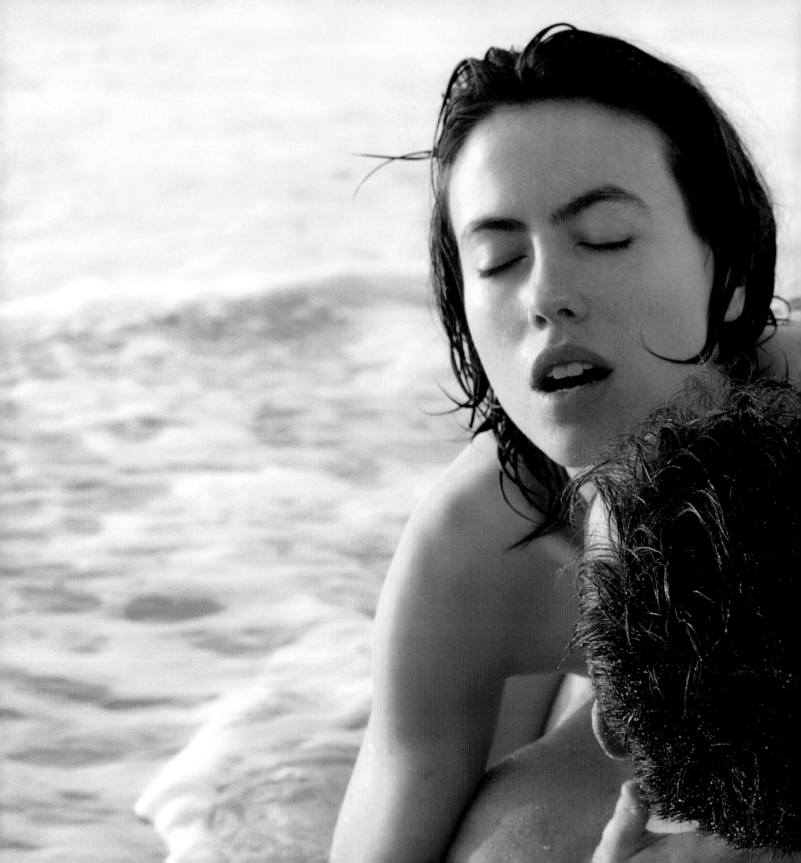

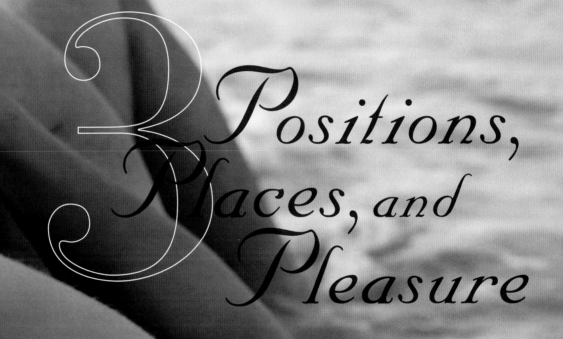

3 Positions, Places, and Pleasure

3 Positions, Places, and Pleasure

AQUATIC SEX IS ALWAYS AN ADVENTURE. Sex in a shower or hot tub is a great way to turn a traditional lovemaking session into an unbridled wet romp, and coupling under a waterfall, on a dock overlooking a lake, or in your pool is the stuff of legends. Aqueous encounters don't require the agility of an acrobat, but there are certain positions and locations that can help make the experience as smooth and sexy as possible.

Poolside Pleasures

Nothing says summer like a glistening swimming pool surrounded by hot bathing suit-clad bodies. Pools are sexy, fun, and playful, and as a result can be the perfect setting for spontaneous wet sex. For those lucky enough to have their own private pool, sex underwater can be a regular occurrence. For the rest of us, acting out our pool fantasies might take a little more creativity. But creativity can always add an extra enticing spark, and plenty of folks are up for the challenge.

When asked to recall their hottest sex ever, a lot of people don't need to think for very long. "For me, it was in a motel pool," says Rina, 28. "My boyfriend and I were driving to Arizona from Los Angeles. We stopped at a super seedy motel one night. The place seemed pretty deserted and there was no one in the pool. We didn't even bother to put bathing suits on—just wrapped ourselves in towels and walked down from our room. It was one of those pools with a kiddie section and low, wide stairs. We were so hot from the drive and feeling the water on my naked skin was one of the best sensations ever. I was leaning back on the steps, and Andre came up between my legs and slid inside me. I normally need more foreplay to get in the mood, but the heat in the air and the cool water covering me just got me really wet. We screwed in that position until I came. Then Andre sat on the edge of the pool while I went down on him."

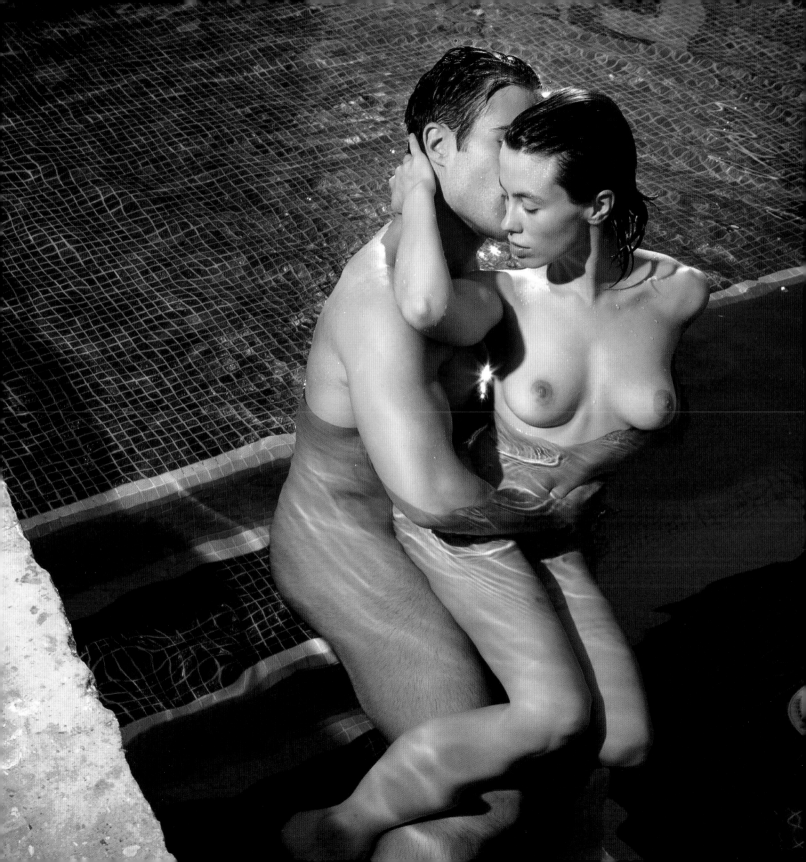

Mina, 29, explains she has always wanted to try sex on a diving board. "I have this image of myself tanning on my back on a diving board when this hottie comes up and pulls off my bathing suit bottoms. He starts licking between my legs, and then I dive into the pool. He follows and we do it underwater." It might not be as hard as Mina thinks to choreograph such an encounter. All she needs is a private pool, a willing partner—and a little balance!

Andy, 29, first had sex in a pool during college. "I was dating a girl whose parents had a pool. She invited me over one weekend when they were out of town. The pool was amazing, kidney-shaped and overlooking a tennis court. We could see the people playing tennis below us, but unless they looked up, they couldn't see us. We had had sex in my dorm room before, but the sex we had in the pool literally blew that out of the water. I felt like I was transitioning from kid stuff to hot adult sex just based on where we were doing it."

The Infinity Pool

Nothing beats out an infinity pool for a sexy swim. Infinity pools create the illusion that water extends to the horizon infinitely. Though the edge of the pool is below the water level, and water spills into a furrowed drain, the visual effect can make the pool's edges seem endless. This is particularly breathtaking when the edge of the pool appears to merge into a larger body of water such as the ocean, or with the sky. For people who love the sense of freedom and the connection with nature that an immense body of water offers, making love in an infinity pool might be one of the most romantic and sensual experiences ever.

WET 'N WILD

Potential Pitfalls of Pool Sex:

- *Slipping.* The pool floor or deck can be slippery. Make sure you are on solid ground before you go to town.

- *Rough edges.* If you are leaning against any part of your pool, diving board, or deck, make sure that you are on a smooth surface. No one likes poolburn on their butt!

- *Bathing suits.* If you plan on taking it all off, make sure you know where it went. Finding your suit at the bottom of the pool can be tricky, especially if you are planning a nighttime session.

- *Family, neighbors, and the lifeguard.* Depending on whether you are using a public or private pool, any one of these interlopers can interrupt your lovemaking. Though many people get off on exhibitionism, having sex in public can actually get you in trouble with the law (or at least nice Mrs. Smith for whom you are cat sitting).

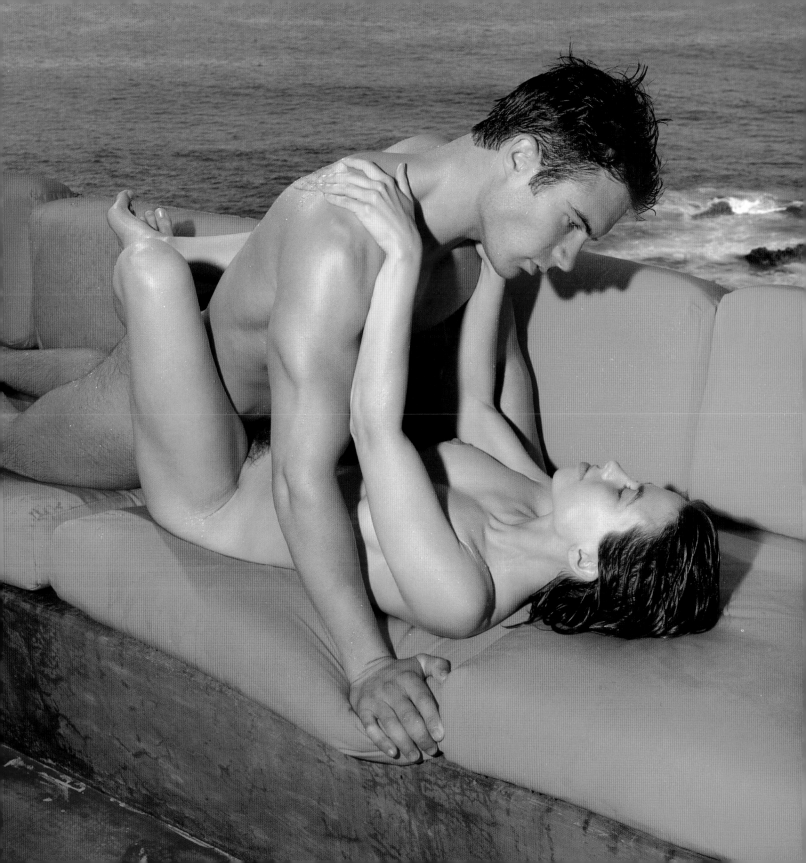

Pool Positions

Try out some of the following perfect pool positions for a wild water romp:

The Straddle

The buoyancy of a pool can help a man hold his partner up even if he doesn't have superhuman upper body strength. For this position, it is best to stay in the shallow end of the pool where it is possible to stand. The man might also want to lean against the wall of the pool for added support. His partner can wrap her legs around his waist as he penetrates her. He will support her weight by keeping his arms under her buttocks. This way it will be easy for the man to help the woman create the perfect rhythm. Alternatively, the woman can use the edge of the pool to help herself slide up and down his shaft as he continues to support her weight.

Diving Board Dynamo

A man holds himself up under the diving board, gripping the sides of the board with each hand. His partner then straddles him with her legs wrapped around his waist as he penetrates her. She holds on to his shoulders or the board for support. Leaning back can help avoid awkward head bumps!

The Ladder Lay

Many pools have vertical ladders with handy bars to grasp. The woman faces the ladder and grabs the bars while her partner enters her from behind. Once he is in position, he can also use the bars for support. For variation, she can place her feet on the bottom rung and stick her butt up in the air. This can help create a doggy style-like experience.

Staircase Sessions

Pools with low, flat staircases can be perfect for a variety of positions. A seated woman can lean back on the stairs with her legs parted as her lover enters her, or a man can sit on the stairs and have his lover climb on top of him. For standing positions, a woman faces the steps and places one foot on the pool floor and one foot two steps up. Using the ledge for support, she can bend forward slightly and enjoy a rear-entry position with ease.

Ledge Licks

Having one partner sit on the edge of the pool is a great way for the swimming partner to get in some good licks and sucks, as the seated partner is in the perfect position to receive oral sex.

A Brief History of the Swimming Pool

People have enjoyed swimming for thousands of years. Ancient Egyptians, Greeks, and Romans were all swimmers. In fact, the Romans are credited with building the first swimming pools and are even reported to have invented a system for heating them. Yet, despite their lengthy history, swimming pools really only took off in the 1800s. By 1837, six indoor pools with diving boards had been built in London, England. Sixty years later, the modern Olympic Games debuted and introduced the idea of swimming races to a vast audience. Swimming became much more fashionable, and as a result, towns and cities all over the world began swimming pool construction.

Of course, pools are more than simply exercise devices. In modern America, the private swimming pool is a site of relaxation, fitness, and in many communities, a status symbol. In his book, *The Springboard in the Pond: An Intimate History of the Swimming Pool*, Thomas A. P. Van Leeuwen explains the backyard swimming pool as a "quintessentially modern and American space, reflecting America's infatuation with hygiene, skin, and recreation." With this in mind, is it really any wonder that so many people find swimming pools the perfect spot for a sexy aquatic romp?

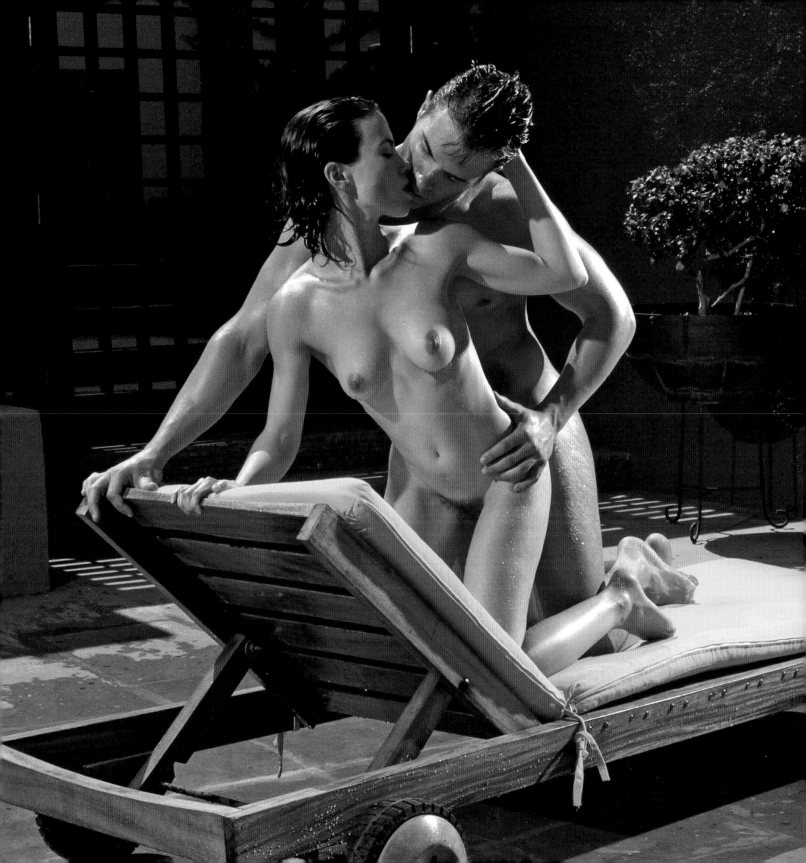

Wet and Steamy Shower Scenarios

Natalia, 41, didn't always enjoy sex in the shower. She says, "Sex in the shower always seemed a little uncomfortable to me. Guys would try to back me against a wall and hold me up. I would do it when a lover wanted to, but it never seemed to go smoothly. Then I met Marco, and the whole experience was totally different. He turned me around and bent me over as the water came down on my back and I loved every minute of it!"

Safe, Sexy Tips for Aquatic Sex

CONDOMS CAN STILL BE USED in or under the water. Unless you have an allergy, it is best to use a latex condom in water. For the 1 to 2 percent of people who are allergic to latex, try a plastic polyurethane condom. Avoid animal skin condoms, which are porous and only offer protection from pregnancy, not infections. Two potential problems you might encounter when using a condom in water are:

• *Lube.* Many condoms come coated with an artificial lubricant. Generally, this lubricant is water based. That's great on dry land, but put a water-based lube in water itself and you will see it simply wash away (much the same way a woman's natural lubrication does). The best thing to do is to use a silicone-based lube. Brands like Bodyfluid, Wet, and Eros all make great silicone lubes. And, unlike oil-based lubes, the silicone varieties are compatible with latex condoms.

• *Slippage.* It is easiest to put on a condom outside of the water where you can see what you are doing and feel that it is on properly. Though condoms are effective in water, they might be more likely to slip off, and you might be less likely to notice this. Regularly check the condom to make sure it is still in place.

Though people often assume that in order to have sex in a shower a man has to be able to hold up his partner, this isn't the case at all. One of the hottest positions for shower sex is a semi-standing doggy style. A woman stays standing and bends forward. She may want to brace herself on the shower wall. From here, her partner can slide into her from behind. A variation on this is to have a woman face the wall and place her foot on the edge of the tub or ledge while bending forward slightly and pushing out her behind. For those who like face-to-face sex, a woman can lean back against the wall and have her partner cradle her leg in his arm. For the very flexible, it may be possible to put your leg on his shoulder. But only try this if it doesn't feel like a strain.

The shower is also a great place for soaking wet oral sex. Either person can kneel on the floor of the shower or tub and use their mouth and tongue to lick and suck a partner. To make this position more comfortable, try placing a folded up towel under your knees or use some tub pillows.

There are countless reasons why shower sex is such a steamy affair. As Jason, 27, explains, "Doing it is the shower intensifies everything. I like to position myself under the stream of water so that I have different sensations all over my body. The water on my back, her mouth on my mouth, and me inside her just makes every nerve ending I have come alive!"

Others cite the quick clean-up, change of scenery, and steamy heat as reasons for the shower appeal. Lance, 34, says, "My girl was really embarrassed to have sex when she had her period. It didn't bother me, but I didn't want to make her uncomfortable. I suggested we do it in the shower, and so that became our monthly ritual." Whatever the reason, plenty of people agree that sex in the shower can't be beat.

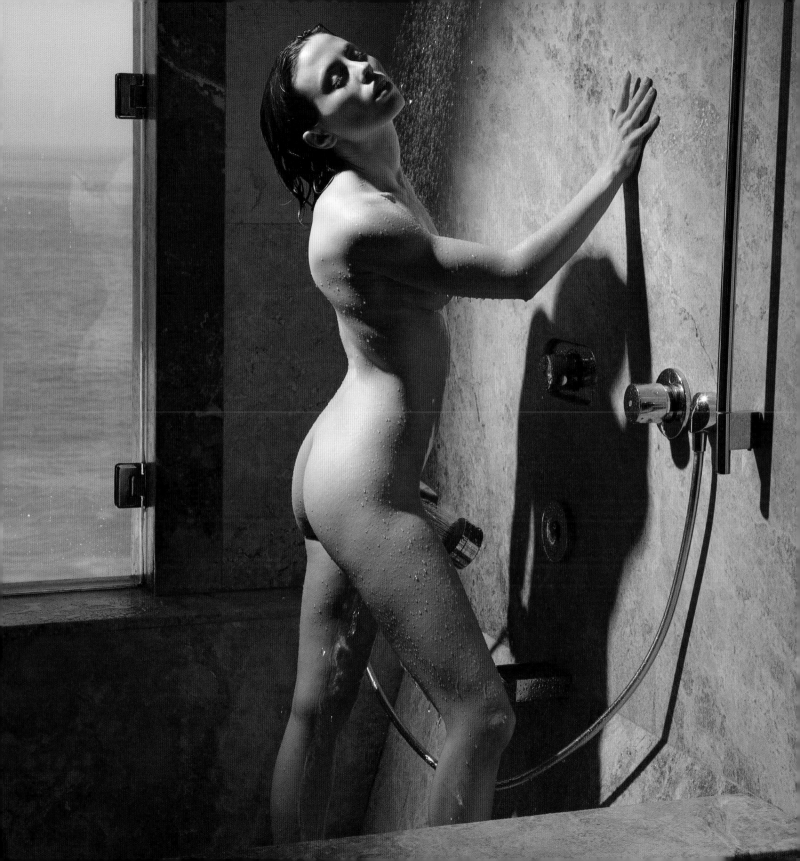

"*My favorite place* to masturbate is in the shower. I love feeling the water spray over my body. When I spread my legs and let the water reach up and down the insides of my thighs, and then move the *shower head spray* directly on my clitoris, *a tingling sensation* shoots straight through my body. I often imagine the hands of my lover caressing me as I move the water stream back and forth over my vagina, my breasts, and my nipples. I always have *multiple orgasms* during these self-touch sessions. It's amazing that just water—a natural element—can create such an electrifying *whole-body experience!*"

—Abby, 28

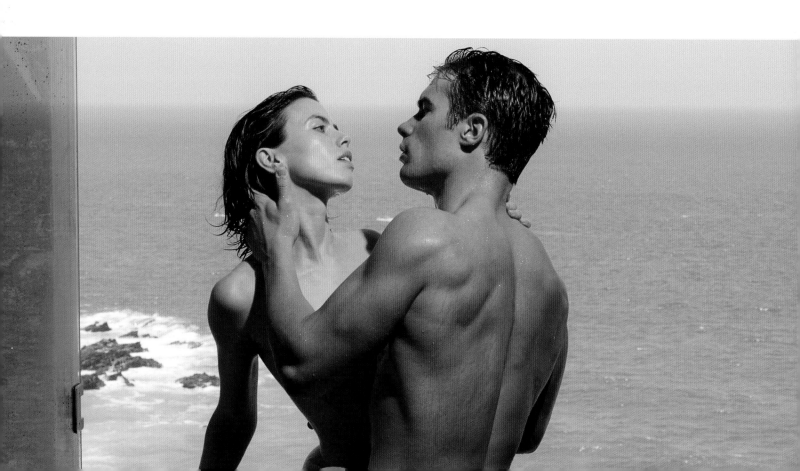

WET 'N WILD

Let's face it, sex can be sloppy. Though plenty of people get off on the sights, smells, and fluids that accompany sex, they're not for everyone. Sex in the shower can be a great way for the hygienically inclined to stop obsessing about mess and start focusing on the action.

Potential Pitfalls of Shower Sex

• *Slipping.* Many showers are slippery. Get a good, secure bath or shower mat. Don't ruin a dripping-wet sex session by banging your head on the faucet as you lose your footing.

• *Cramped space.* Stall showers don't offer a lot of room for movement. Rather than trying to turn yourself into a human pretzel, it might be best to leave the actual screwing for a setting with a little more space. Instead, take advantage of the closeness of your lover's wet slick body and how good it feels to slide up and down each other. Let the excitement build up for what is about to come.

• *Height.* Some positions just aren't going to work as well if there are great height disparities. Don't injure yourself attempting something that your body cannot achieve. There are plenty of amazing positions that *will* work, so focus on those instead.

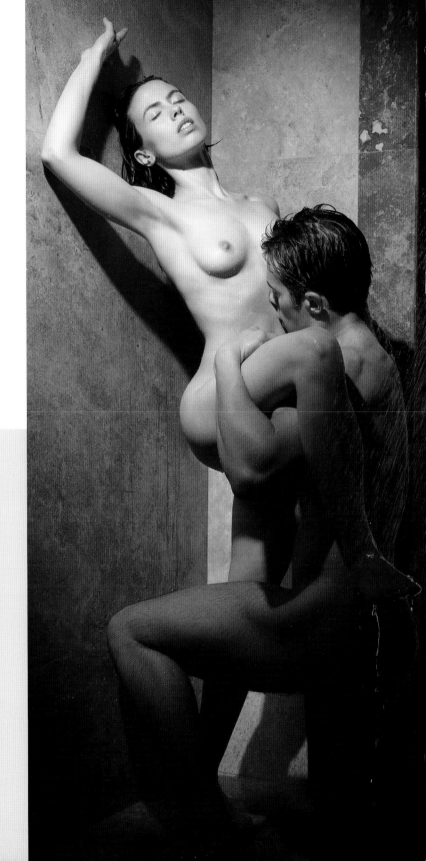

WET 'N WILD

Try shaving your partner in the tub or shower. A woman's legs, a man's face, and even the pubic area can all be treated to a sensual shave by a lover. Make sure to use a fresh razor and plenty of lather as you go. Then luxuriate as smooth skin begins to emerge beneath your fingers.

Bathtub Booty

Unless you have a particularly large bathtub, sex with a partner in such a confined space can be tricky, but it is by no means impossible. Delores, 39, has had plenty of tub sex with scintillating results. In particular, she recommends doggy style. "I like to get on my hands and knees and have my man do me from behind in the tub. We have a thick mat on the bottom of the tub, so it doesn't hurt to be in that position. A few times we tried it missionary style, but there wasn't quite enough room for his legs, and we realized doing it from behind worked better." Other good bathtub positions include:

The X-tra

He lies back in the tub with his legs apart and his head at one end of the tub. She lies on her back with her head at the other end and lowers herself onto his penis. This position is great for gentle rocking, but not ideal for hard thrusting because the man's penis will be at an angle.

Sit 'n Splash

He sits in the middle of the tub with his legs stretched in front of him. She straddles him and slides into a sitting position on his penis, and then wraps her legs around his waist.

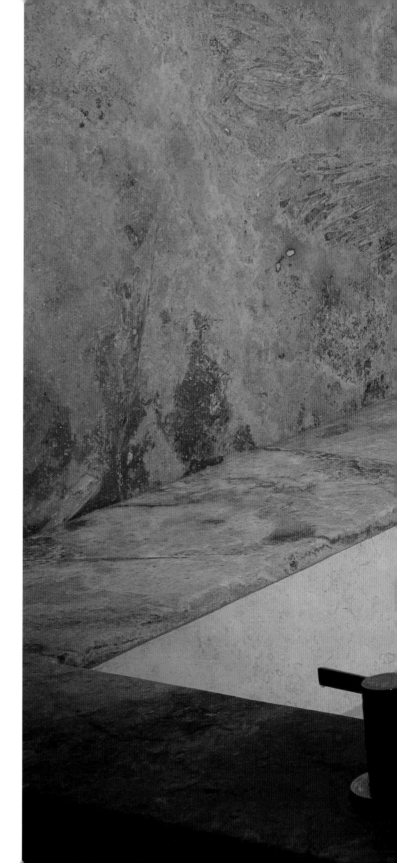

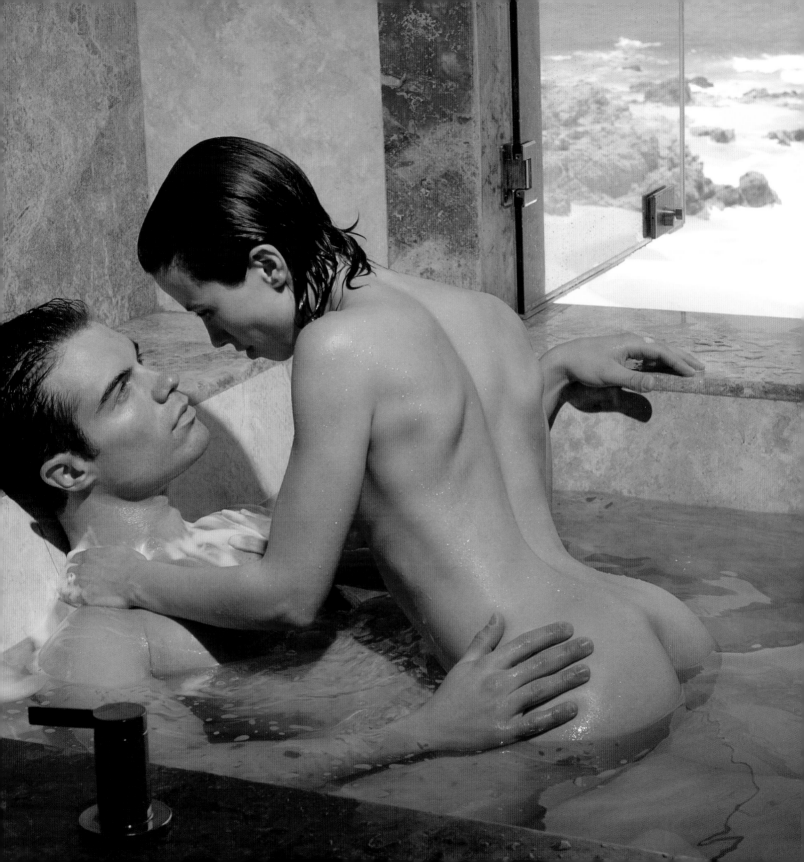

Backward Booty

He leans back in the tub. She squats over him, facing the opposite side of the tub. After sliding his penis inside of her, she can slowly lean forward and rest her arms on or between his legs.

Sensual Soaking

For those who enjoy the tub's more sensuous properties, there are many options. Dave, 43, enjoys soaking in the tub with his wife. "I love taking a bath with Melody. Even though our tub is incredibly small, I like to lean against the back and have her recline on me between my legs. That way I can press myself against her and cup her breasts. The whole experience is relaxing and makes me feel close to her without having to have sex."

Tubs are also great for the exhibitionists and voyeurs among us. Many people love watching a partner bathe and get off on helping out from the sidelines. "I don't *really* need help washing my back," says Suli, 22, "but I always call my boyfriend when I'm taking a bath to do it for me. Sometimes he'll ask if I need help washing anywhere else and I'll tell him I'm probably dirty from all the sex we had earlier. If I'm lucky, I'll get washed down below too!" Whether you are simply observing or actually lending a hand, there are few other events that make watching from a dry vantage point so enticing.

Of course, the thought of soaking in a bubble-filled tub or trailing a finger down a sweetie's soap-covered torso will be much more appealing if the rest of the room feels equally romantic. Luckily, the bathroom can be turned into a love nest without too much effort, and setting the stage for erotic encounters with lighting, music, scented candles, and bubble bath are great ways to transform the spot where you brush your teeth into your own private fantasy world. Keep the room warm, turn the lights down low, and you'll be amazed at the change in atmosphere a few minutes of preparation can achieve.

WET 'N WILD

Our olfactory senses play a crucial role in arousal. Scent your bathwater with delicious-smelling essential oils like lavender, jasmine, or orange. Drop in slices of apple or rose petals to complete your sensual soak.

Bathtub Games

Romance is not always what's in the air, sometimes fun is. The bathtub is a great place to splash and play and explore a whole range of sudsy, sexy fun. Try out some of these ideas:

• *Bathtub Love.* This bath time game is a novelty item for adults made up of ten naughty *bath bubbles.* Each plastic bubble contains four different instructions inside, such as "kiss nipples" or "give oral sex." Pick out one bubble and one instruction at random, then follow.

• Remember, toys aren't only for kids. A waterproof vibrator can be the perfect way to get off while soaking. Use your vibe alone or when sharing the tub. You can also ask a lover to help you out, whether he is in the tub with you or not. For added enjoyment, try a waterproof vibrating bath sponge, which you can find at most sex toy shops or online sites.

• Hit the toy store for some nonpermanent fingerpaints. Cover your lover's body with your most fanciful designs, then stand up and turn on the shower for a multicolored rinse.

WET 'N WILD

If your bathtub isn't big enough for two, it might be just as fun to have one person stay tubside, freeing up space for more extensive teasing, tickling, and tantalizing.

Hot Tub Heaven

Hot tubs first emerged in America in the late 1950s when soldiers returning from the Second World War constructed their own, having experienced *ofuros* (wooden tubs used for communal bathing) in Japan. By the 1970s, hot tubs were found around the country, and they quickly became a mainstay of the freewheeling party set. Though hot tubs are sold on their relaxing and therapeutic properties, they also hold great sex appeal. Warm, bubbly, and decadent, hot tubs present countless possibilities. Trevor, 42, calls his hot tub *The Seducer*. "I say that as a joke, but it's true that after a soak in the tub more than a few women have ended up in my bed." An outdoor hot tub on a cold night can be all that is needed to get the blood flowing. Hot tubs are more likely to be found in someone's home than are swimming pools, and as a result they can offer an extra degree of privacy for the aquatic sex adventurer.

Sultry, Sexy, and Soothing Tub Reads for Liquid Leisure

Whether you are soaking alone or with a lover, nothing is sexier than a hot bathtub read. Try running a steaming bubble bath for you and your special someone and then spice up the situation by sensuously reading a few choice passages from your favorite erotica novel. Below are a few choice picks to get you started.

Aqua Erotica: 18 Stories for a Steamy Bath by Mary Anne Mohanraj offers erotic water-themed tales that will get your heart racing. From sexy hot tub parties to underwater artistic endeavors, this book drips with sensual stories. An added bonus: It's waterproof!

For sexy, nonaquatic reads, check out books like *The Story of O* by Pauline Reage, *The Sleeping Beauty Trilogy* by Anne Rice, *Taboo: Forbidden Fantasies for Couples* by Violet Blue, or *Heat Wave: Sizzling Sex Stories* by Alison Tyler.

Potential Bathtub Blunders

• Porcelain is hard. Be careful not to bash your head or elbow on the side of a tub when maneuvering into position.

• Many bath products can irritate the delicate skin of the vulva and vagina. Try to use hypo-allergenic products.

• Don't do anything that could submerge your head, and be careful not to accidentally push a partner's head underwater.

WET 'N WILD

For a truly sexy soak, consider what you sip. In a hot tub, something light and cold, like a crisp glass of white wine, bubbling champagne, an icy gin and tonic, or a frozen margarita, can be a nice prelude to a sexy session.

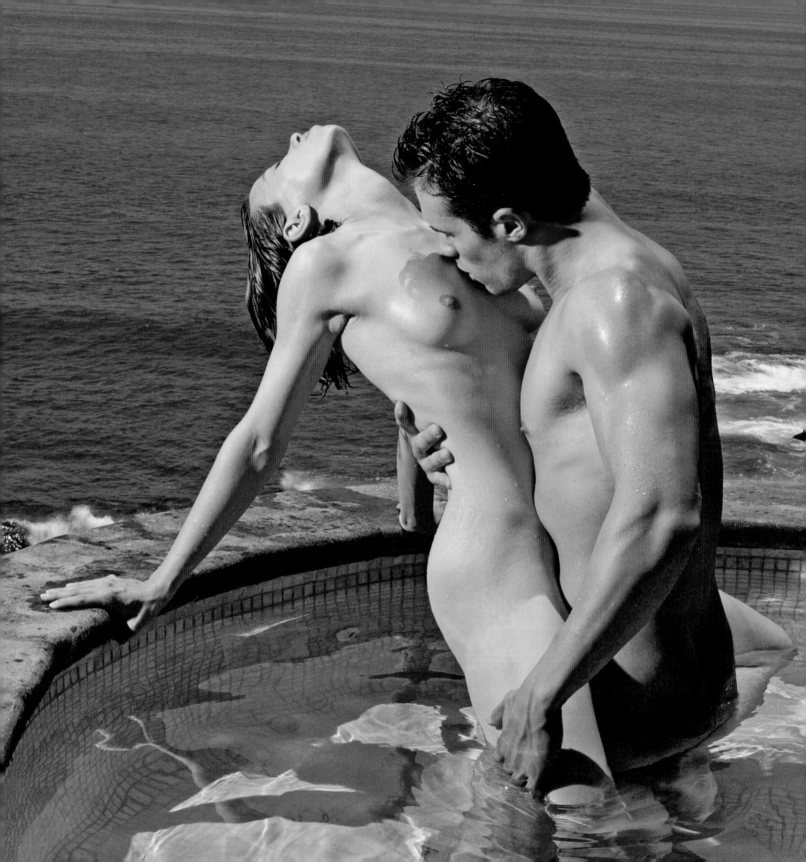

Hot Positions for Hot Tub Sex

For those who want to leave the bed out of sex, here are some tried and tested positions for hot tub lovemaking:

The Straddle

He sits on the bench facing into the tub. She faces him and kneels with her legs on either side of his before lowering herself onto his penis. She can use the edge of the tub for balance and to help push herself up and down his shaft.

Backward Straddle

He sits on the bench facing into the tub. She straddles him, also facing forward. This position is great because neither partner has to worry about bumping knees against the tub's wall. It also allows the man to easily reach forward to caress his partner's breasts or clitoris.

Modified Missionary

She sits on the bench, and her man stands between her legs facing her. He squats slightly and enters her. The buoyancy of the water can help the woman float and the man can support her by placing his hands under her bottom.

Half-doggy

She stands in the tub or kneels on the bench and supports herself on the ledge of the tub. He then enters her from behind. When standing it can be pleasurable to place one leg on the bench for deeper penetration.

The Jet Stream

The force of water from a hot tub jet has sent many cleverly positioned woman over the edge. You might want to try some of the above positions with added water jet placement to see how intense the effect becomes!

Potential Hot Tub Hazards

• Chemicals in hot tubs can irritate the genitals. If, after a soak or sex session, you feel uncomfortable down below, get checked out.

• Depending on where your hot tub is located, you may or may not be providing a show to anyone who cares to watch.

• Very powerful jets might provide too much pressure for direct contact with your nether regions.

• Kneeling on a hard surface can cause discomfort and bruising. Bring a bath pillow!

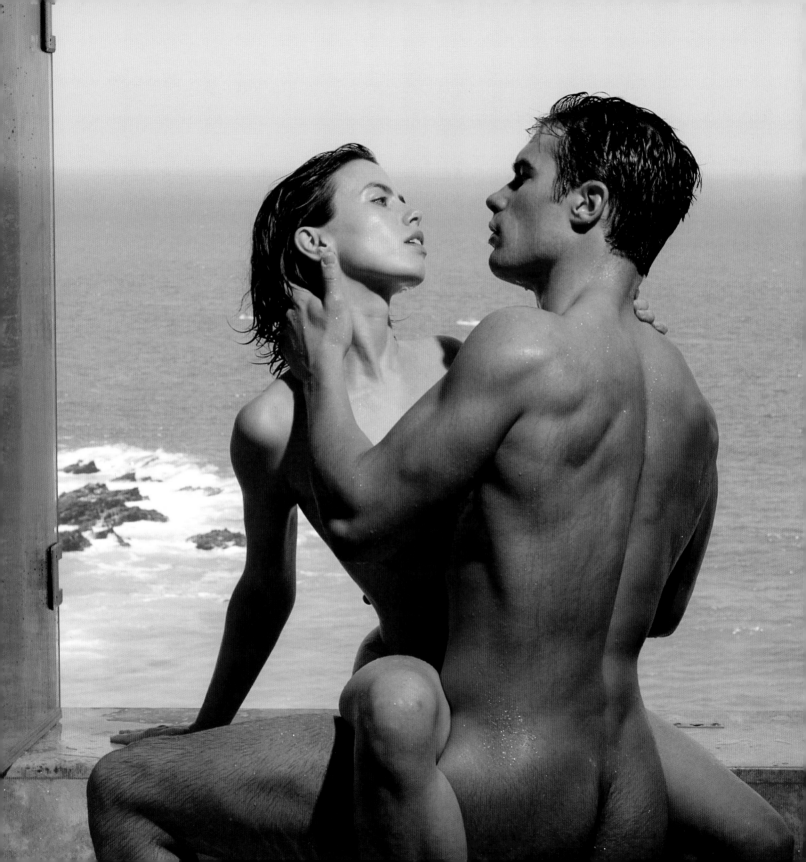

"I always thought hot tub sex sounded a little cliché. However, that was before I had actually had it. My wife and I were away on a ski vacation and decided to take dip in the *hot tub to relax* our sore muscles. Well, it ended up being one of the most *erotic experiences* I've had with her in a long time. Being submerged in bubbling, hot water, with the cold air outside, was *such a turn-on* for me that I had to take her right there in the hot tub. Needless to say, we spent our après-ski in there for the next week!"

—Joel, 35

Why Wash?

Having a bathtub or shower in one's home is something we all take for granted, but it wasn't too long ago that bathing was done either at a public location—with a sponge and a bucket—or not at all. In fact, at different points throughout history, Western Europeans believed bathing to be unappealing, and even unhygienic! Napoleon Bonaparte is famous for writing a letter to his wife Josephine asking her to refrain from bathing in the weeks leading up to his return home from battle. Though this might seem odd and unpleasant to our contemporary understanding of sexiness and cleanliness, throughout history many people have appreciated a lover's natural scent and muskiness. Regular washing can dilute these odors and mask pheromones, the hormonal secretions that are released from our bodies to act as natural sex signals. Though you may smell as sweet as a freshly plucked rose after a good scrub, your lover might actually be craving the animalistic odor that just trickled down the drain. Who knows, maybe Napoleon was on to something . . .

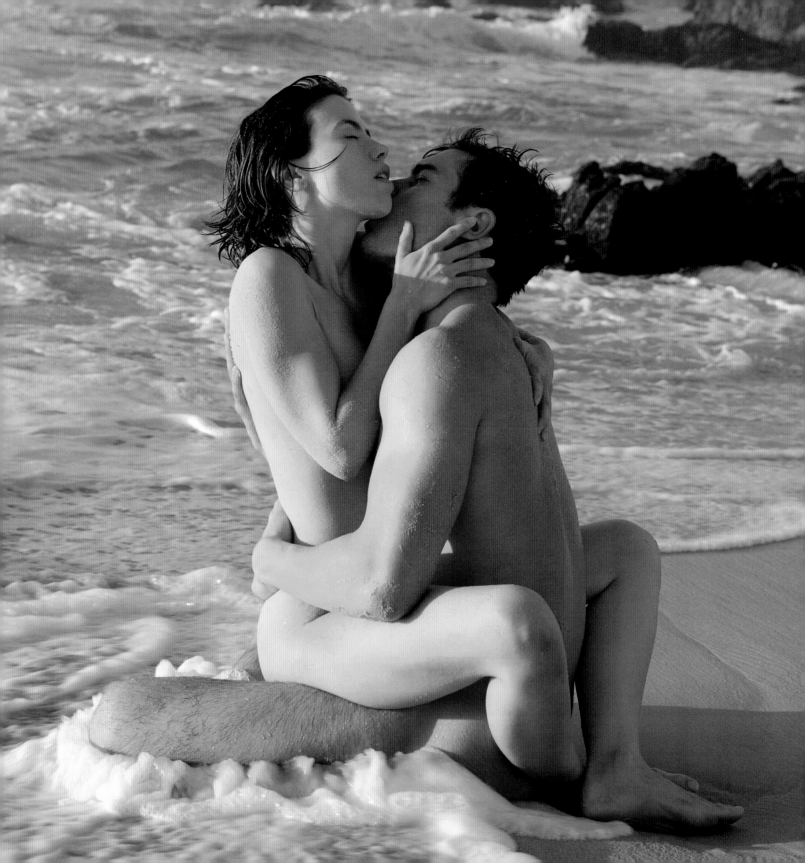

"My husband and I were on our honeymoon in the Caribbean, and one day I was swimming, and he came up behind me and I could tell he was hard. He convinced me to swim out to the sandbar, and *we had sex right there,* with our bodies *submerged underwater.* It was such an erotic experience—the wetness, being weightless in the beautiful azure water—that *I came right away,* even though it usually takes me awhile. It was one of the most memorable parts of our trip!"

—Jessica, 29

Oceanic Adventures

When it comes to romance, nothing beats sitting on the beach with your honey and watching the sun set over the ocean. So is it any wonder that sex under these circumstances is so appealing? The sounds of seagulls flying overhead and waves crashing around you can be aphrodisiac enough to get your blood flowing and your heart racing. Couple that with a sexy someone lounging on a blanket next to you, and your night is set. Laila, 24, enjoys sex play in the ocean, but only under the cover of darkness. "I know some people will have sex in the water during the day, but to me it is a nighttime activity. I like the fact that people might be close by—sitting on the beach or even in the water—but don't know what is going on a few feet away from them." Night or day, sex in the sea offers numerous possibilities.

For sex on the beach, bring a few supplies along. The most crucial one is a large blanket. No matter how much you love the feeling of sand on your back, you aren't going to like it much when it gets into your most intimate places. A second blanket can also be helpful, both for privacy and for warmth. Beaches can get chilly after the sun sets. If you don't come prepared, doing it doggy style is probably your best bet, as this position keeps your nether regions as far from the sand as possible.

That said, in the middle of the day, the scorching sun might do a number on your bare bottom or boobs. If these places haven't seen the light of day since you were a naked two-year-old, don't forget to slather on some SPF 45 before you do your business!

Sex in the ocean itself can be extremely erotic. Many people enjoy the connection to water. As Samantha, 37, explains, "Water is so sensual. To be enveloped in it makes me feel connected to nature and to my partner in a way that I never experience when I make love in a bed." One of the most appealing things about the ocean is that, unlike pools, showers, or tubs, you are not bound by walls. The ocean is vast, expansive, and open. As amazing a rush as this can be, it can also make it a little more challenging to find comfortable positions for sex. One of the best ones is the **straddle**. Using the buoyancy of the water, the man holds the woman under her buttocks as she straddles him and wraps her legs around his waist. Planting your feet firmly in the sand can help keep you stable and balanced.

Amazing oceanic sex can also be done at the water's edge, lying in the sand, missionary position. Unlike the dry variety, damp sand will be less likely to work its way into your most intimate parts, and even if it does, the effect of your lover's thrusts combined with waves crashing over you might just make the experience worthwhile.

Oceanic Sex Positions

The Cradle
Partners stand facing each other. He holds one of her legs in his arm and then slides into her. The water will help her stay buoyant and keep you both balanced. This position allows couples to kiss and gaze into each other's eyes. And if you take a tumble, so what? That might just add to the experience.

The Shallow Doggy
Doing it doggy style is a great option for shallow water. A woman can get on all fours while her man positions himself between her legs from behind. From this position, he can reach forward to touch her breasts or her clitoris, and she can reach back to caress his balls. Just make sure not to take in a mouth full of saltwater as you cry out in ecstasy!

The Buoy Bang
Swim over to a buoy. She holds onto the buoy with both hands while he enters her from behind. Guys should make sure to use the buoy and not their lover's shoulders for support. In your excitement, you don't want to inadvertently push your honey under.

Pier Pleasures
A pier is an excellent oceanic prop—as long as it is free of barnacles. Have the woman bend forward holding onto one of the pier's posts. Grabbing the post or holding her shoulders for support, the man can enter her from behind. Sex under a pier allows you a degree of privacy and can be a great place to get the full effect of crashing waves.

When having sex in the ocean, it is always helpful to look for props. Piers, docks, rafts, and smooth flat rocks can all help you come up with creative new ways to get hot and heavy.

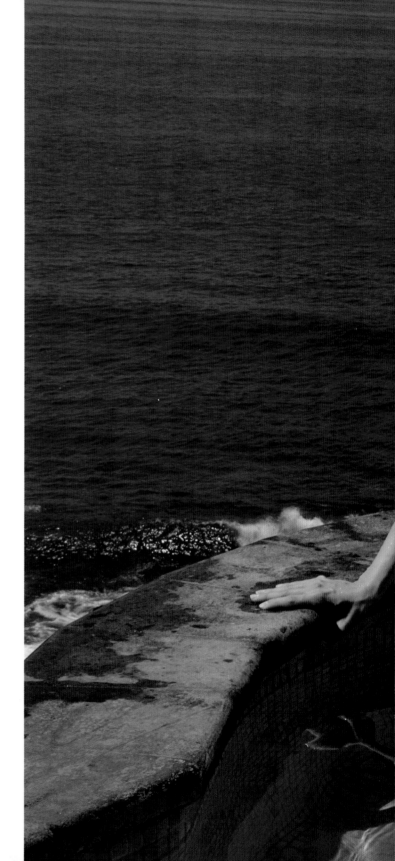

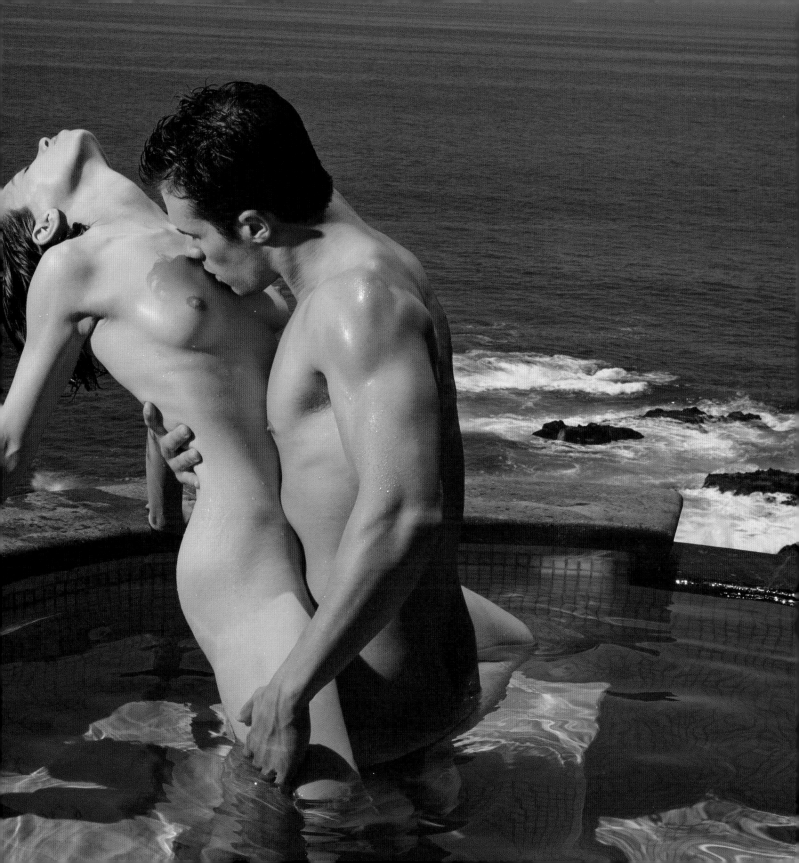

WET 'N WILD

Water offers amazing sensations of flotation and weightlessness, but because it is so buoyant, it can be tough to achieve the forceful thrust of sex on dry land. Consider using your oceanic setting for some hot foreplay, complete with groping, nibbling, and some serious kissing before heading back for a sexy session on the beach.

Potential Pitfalls of Oceanic Sex

• For most people, sex in the ocean is hot and passionate. However, for a few women, seawater can cause vaginal irritations. If after a steamy session you develop itching, burning, or discomfort, see your healthcare provider to make sure everything is under control.

• Avoid positions that can force sand inside delicate body parts. For beach banging, bring a large towel or blanket.

• Try not to gulp down the salty stuff. When ingested, seawater can make you sick.

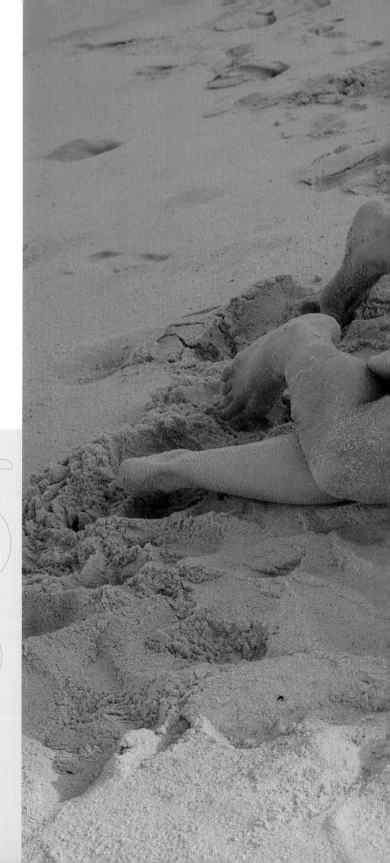

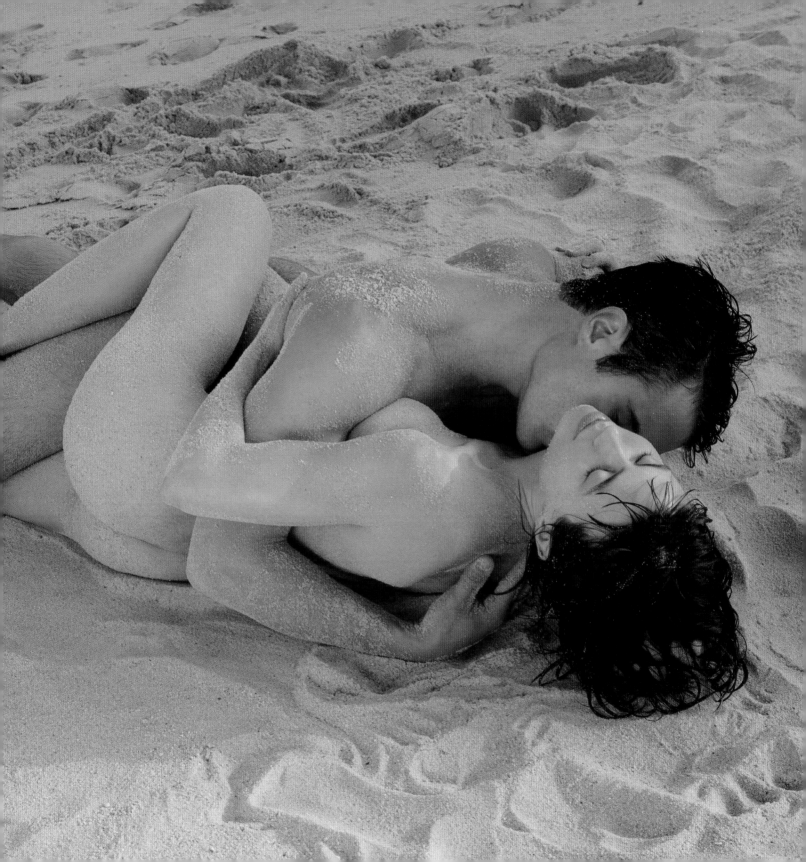

Vacation Variations

Vacations are the perfect time for exploration and adventure. Out of your natural element and free from prying eyes, vacationing allows you to tap into previously unknown aspects of your sexuality and pursue them with abandon. Whether you are exploring with your spouse or lover, or having a steamy affair with a complete stranger, vacations let you try on a different sexual persona, and one you just might be reluctant to give up once the sun, sand, and sea are only distant memories!

For those of us who don't live in the tropics, beach vacations can be an easy fantasy to turn into reality. Mick, from the Northeast, tries to get to a hot spot at least once a year. "The sex I have on vacation is different than the sex I have at home. My wife and I would never go to our local park to screw, but for some reason if we're on a beach in the Caribbean, it is much more likely to end up happening. When we were in Hawaii, last winter, I think we had sex every day, though rarely in the hotel room."

WET 'N WILD

Everyone takes vacation photos, but why not snap a couple of sexy pics of your honey in an exotic location? If you are nervous about having the photos discovered, you can always email the shots to yourself and have a saucy reminder of your holiday waiting for you when you get home.

Allison, 36, has long harbored a fantasy that she hopes to make a reality one day. "If there is any one place I want to have sex, it would be under a waterfall. I picture myself standing under the water. A man comes up behind me and takes off my bikini top as the water crashes over us. Then he takes off my bottom and we stand under the water making love."

Though tropical vacations allow for hot beach sex, there are other ways to incorporate your love of liquid lust into your travel plans. Many a hiker has cooled off after a long trek by plunging nude into a mountain stream. And countless campers have enjoyed lakeside lovemaking. Sanjay, 31, is one of them. When camping, he seeks out secluded lakeside spots to pitch his tent both for the solitude and the sexiness. "I love going camping with women I'm dating. For me, if a woman isn't into the outdoors, I know it won't last long. One of the things I think it the sexiest is to wake up early in the morning and jump into the water naked with my girl. It makes me feel invigorated and ready for the day." Nature can be an intense aphrodisiac. If you get turned on by the ocean and the tropics, you might also find a wet woodsy setting to be to your liking.

Getting away from your usual routine is a great way to explore your wild (and wet) sides. Miranda, 31, recalls letting loose on vacation. "I was very prim and proper in my twenties and I dressed very conservatively. I've always been shy about my body, so I never wanted to draw attention to it. One spring I got dragged to my cousin's bachelorette party in Miami. My cousin and I are very different. I'll be drinking a glass of red wine, and she'll be lying on the bar as guys lick tequila off her chest. I knew her party would be pretty wild, but I figured I would just leave early. I ended up staying until the bitter end, and getting talked into a wet t-shirt contest! I don't know if I'll ever do that again, but I don't regret it. It was exciting to feel sexy and know that I was turning people on." Things that you never thought yourself

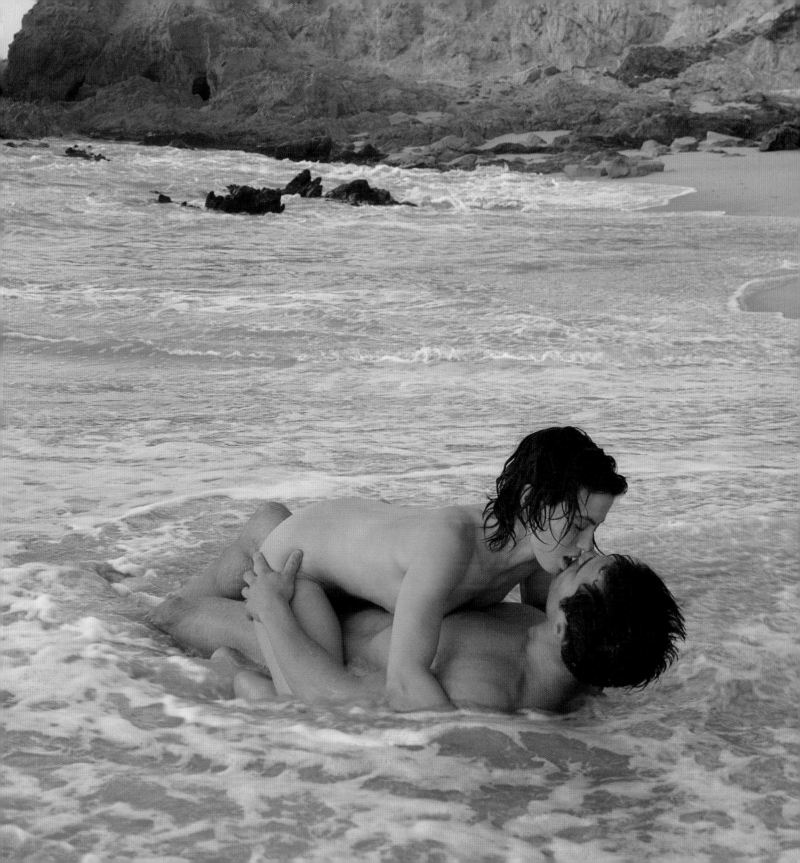

capable of at home, like participating in wet t-shirt contests, having sex in a public pool, or rolling around with a stranger you just met on a foreign beach, can all come to life on vacation.

One popular vacation exploit is exploring you exhibitionist side. When no one you know from home is likely to see your naughty bits, exposing them can seem less daunting! Exhibitionism is the desire to display naked parts of the body to others or to have others watch you engage in sex acts. There are many reasons people enjoy exhibiting themselves. Some crave attention, others are proud of their bodies and sexuality. At times, exhibitionism can help a person validate his or her sexual desires or sense of sex appeal. Though some people enjoy the thrill of shocking unsuspecting passersby with their antics, contrary to what we may think, most exhibitionists are not simply sleazy flashers in trench coats. In fact, plenty of perfectly normal and healthy people have an exhibitionist streak within.

Many aquatic sex fantasies have an exhibitionist element to them. The swimming pool, beach, or boat that you are envisioning for a hot sex session, may derive some of its appeal from the fact that it is a semi-public place where you could potentially be caught in the act. Of course, getting caught in the act isn't always what it is cracked up to be. Having sex, (and even being nude) in public is generally illegal. Additionally, as sexy as it might be for you to have sex in front of other people, those other people might not be as excited by the idea, and often will be downright uncomfortable or offended. Still, there are plenty of safe and fun ways for exhibitionists to show their stuff. Here are a few tips:

· Leave the underwear at home. One of the easiest ways to exhibit yourself is to do so secretly. Only you and your sweetie need to know that nothing lies between your clothes and your flesh. The experience of walking around without that extra layer beneath your clothes can be quite a thrill.

· Try out a super-skimpy bathing suit. Dental floss can be good for more than just your teeth.

· Visit a nude beach. Though most naturists are adamant about the fact that nudity to them is not sexual, a nude beach is a perfectly acceptable place to show your stuff. Just make sure you don't cross any boundaries or make unwanted sexual advances.

· Seek out like-minded people. Don't try to talk an uncomfortable partner into public sex. Doing so will most likely not be fun for either of you. If this is really important to you, you might be better off with someone who shares your desires

· If you decide to have sex in public, always make sure to have something available for a quick cover-up. A wrap or blanket can be a handy tool.

· Swing clubs and sex parties are the best place to display your goods among people who want to look at them. If wetness is your thing, do a bit of research to find groups that offer pool or hot tub parties. If you can't find any clubs in your area that meet your needs, consider starting one yourself.

· Take a sexy vacation to a resort like Jamaica's *Hedonism*, which caters to exhibitionism and nudity.

· Use the Internet. The Web is crawling with amateurs and professionals alike who enjoy displaying themselves. If you choose to go this route, make sure you are comfortable with possible unwanted attention, or being discovered by a boss or family member. And always take proper safety precautions by never posting your name or contact information along with any pictures.

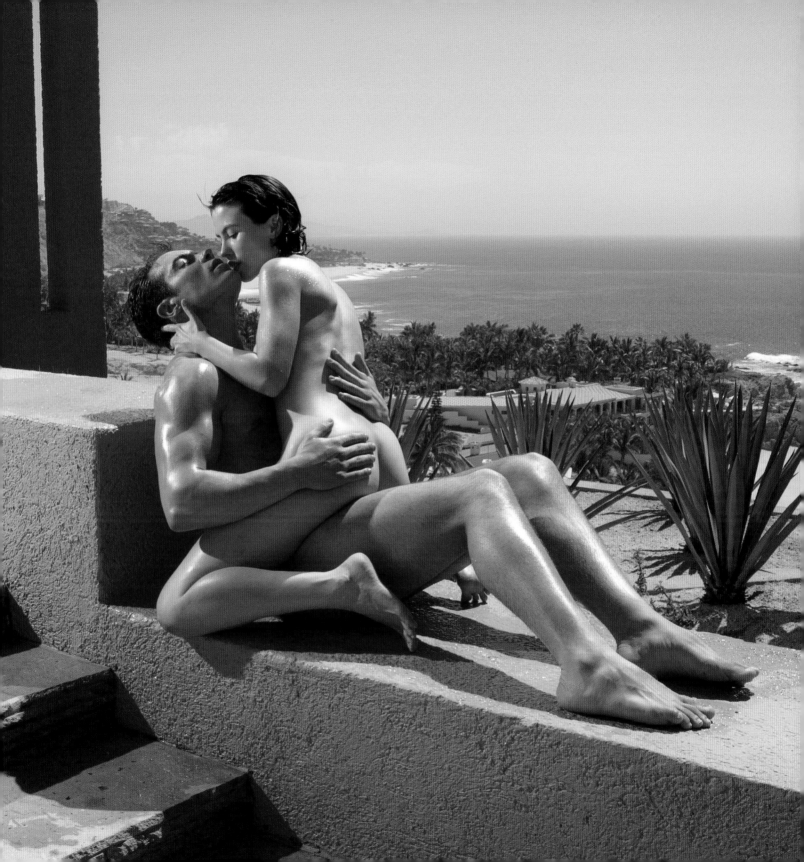

Melanie's First Time

"I was a virgin until I was twenty-six. I wasn't waiting for marriage, I'm just very shy. As a result, I didn't date a lot in college or after. Then I was sent to a conference in Australia for work, and I decided to make a vacation out of it as well. I had never traveled by myself before and was very nervous about meeting new people, but on my first night off, I forced myself to go to a restaurant on the beach that looked very romantic. I got a table for one, and a very cute guy as my waiter. He was extremely attentive and sweet, and we chatted and flirted throughout the entire meal. Then I did something I never would have done at home. I asked him when he got off work that night. His eyes lit up and he stuttered a little and asked if I would like to come back at eleven when his shift ended. I did, and we walked down to the beach and sat by the water as the waves came in. I had never had a date like it. We laughed and flirted and kissed, and I even told him I was a virgin. I asked if he would like to be my first and if he would take me right there on the beach by the water. It was almost as if being on the other side of the world allowed me to tap into a part of myself I didn't know existed. I'm really glad that my first sexual experience happened the way it did. I felt in control and confident and sexy in a way I think I wouldn't have under any circumstances back in the States."

Steamy Hot Springs

A hot spring occurs when warm or hot groundwater regularly bubbles from the earth in a particular spot. Often boasting a high mineral content, hot springs have long been sought out for their therapeutic and healing properties and can be found across North America, as well as around the world in countries as diverse as Iceland, New Zealand, and Japan. Because resorts and spas are often built around hot springs, they can make for a relaxing and romantic getaway. Marcella, 28, recalls her honeymoon spent at a hot spring resort. "Jason and I were trying to figure out what to do on our honeymoon. I wanted to go somewhere tropical and beachy, but we only had a weekend to spare. We ended up at a lovely hot spring resort in Colorado. There were indoor and outdoor pools. It was winter, and we would race to the outdoor ones in our suits and towels, jump in, and then when we were done, race back inside. We spent half the time running through the cold laughing hysterically and the other half lounging in the water."

Nick, 29, has taken lovers to hot spring getaways on a few occasions. "I've been to two or three really rustic hot spring locations with women I was involved with," he says. "I took my girlfriend to one place during the off-season. It was very bare bones: wood cabins, a canteen, and, of course, the springs. There was hardly anyone there, and we would wake up, soak in one of the springs and then, feeling completely relaxed, spend the rest of the morning in bed, before hitting the springs again. It was an amazing cycle of sex and relaxation. I don't think we were dry for most of the weekend."

Though not hailed for their aphrodisiac properties to the same extent that oysters and Spanish fly are, natural phenomena, like hot springs, often have the greatest effect on the libido. When we are surrounded by comfort and beauty, feeling healthy and relaxed, it is that much easier to let ourselves sink into the kind of effortless sex that can be hard to achieve while leading a hectic life back home.

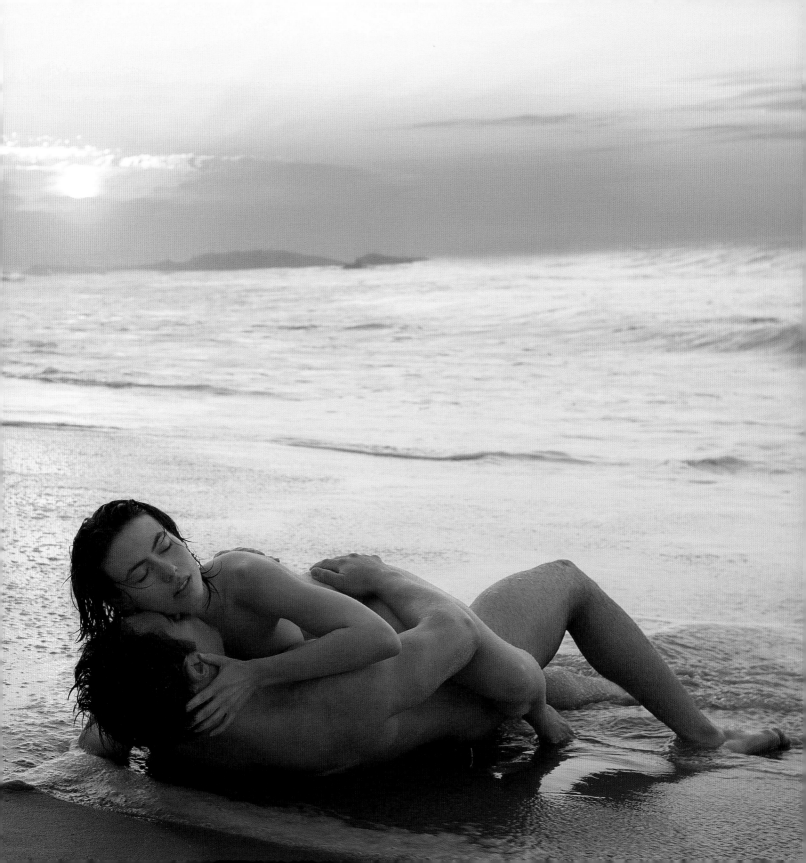

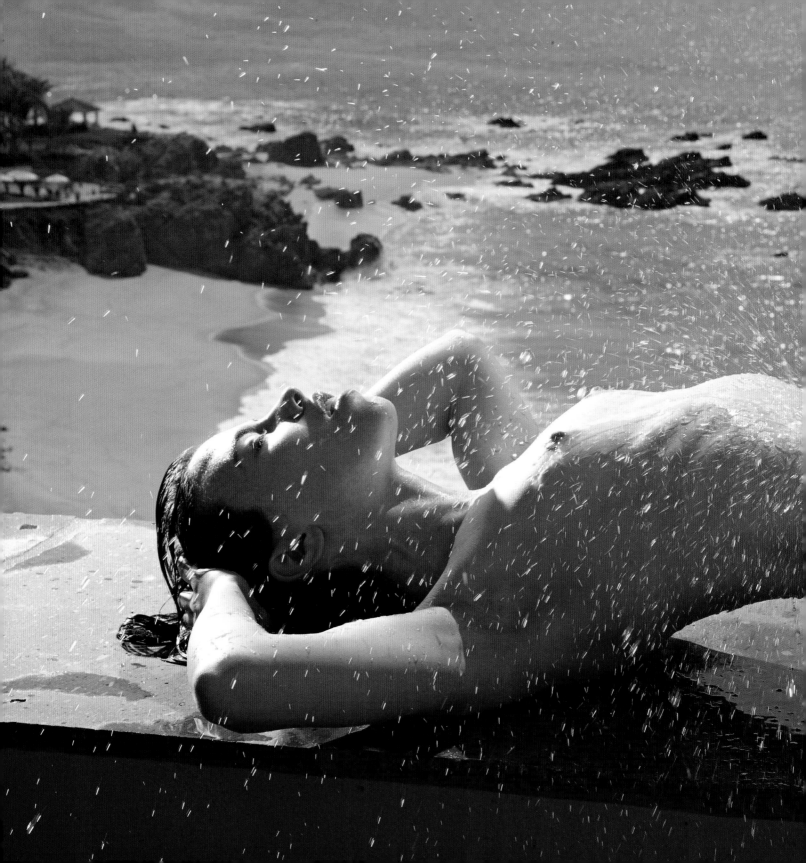

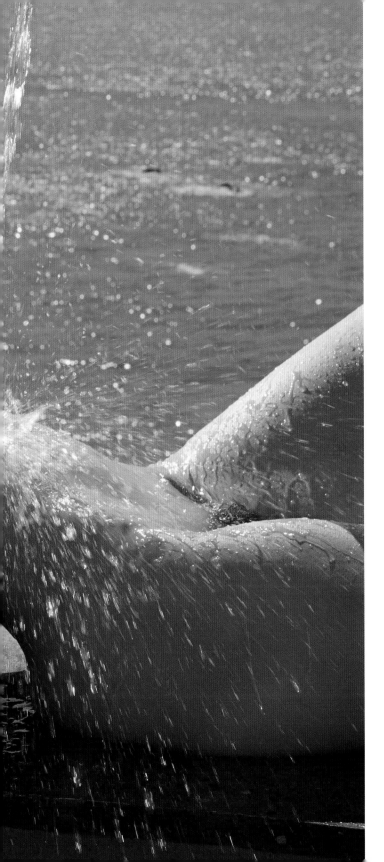

Assessing Arousal

Whether you are breathing heavily on a beach in Bali or luxuriating alone in your bathtub, the presence of water is undeniably sexy. Water is the source of all life on earth, so is it really any wonder that it possesses the power to arouse us to unbelievable heights? Depending on the circumstances, wet sex play can as easily be romantic and sensuous as it can be naughty and adventurous. Expressing our aqueous sexuality allows myriad possibilities for sexual fun and exploration. Though not every suggestion in this chapter is going to be your thing, trying out a few different ideas can really get the creative juices flowing. Who knows, you might be surprised to find out how much you enjoy sexy games, making love in your pool, or languishing in the tub for an hour with your naughtiest book of erotica.

Underwater Hotels

For those who want to try their hand at a nautical version of the "Mile-High Club," spending a night at an underwater hotel could be just the thing.

In Florida, check into Jules' Undersea Lodge. Originally used as a research laboratory to explore the continental shelf off the coast of Puerto Rico, Jules' has served as an underwater hotel for the past twenty years. To reach the hotel, guests need to scuba dive 21 feet beneath the surface of the sea and swim through tropical mangroves. Once inside, they are treated to many of the comforts of a regular hotel as they gaze out the windows at sea creatures floating by. The hotel even offers wedding and honeymoon packages that promise "all of the romance and adventure of an underwater wedding combined with the comfort and convenience of a dry setting."

Other underwater hotels are currently being planned in places as far reaching as China, Dubai, and the Bahamas.

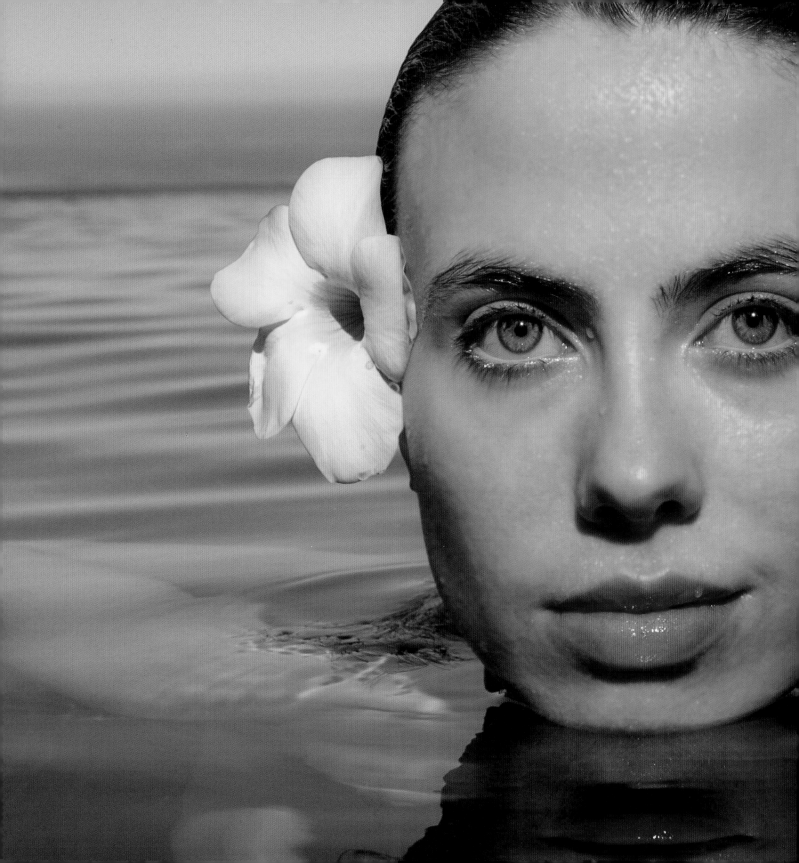

4 Solo Sailing

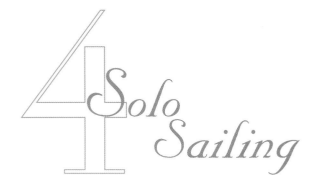

4 Solo Sailing

WHETHER YOU ARE COUPLED OR SINGLE, solo sex can open the doors to countless possibilities for pleasure and exploration. Touching yourself is a great way to release sexual tension. It is also a fantastic method for learning about your most personal turn-ons. Not only do solitary explorations keep boredom at bay on otherwise lonely nights, but the best lovers are often those who are most intimately acquainted with their own bodies and can show a partner exactly how they like to be caressed and stimulated. For water lovers, solo sex offers numerous possibilities, from sexy soaks in the tub to heating up over a naughty aquatic flick. When it comes to getting wet, there is no need to wait for a partner before diving in!

Aquatic Fantasies

If there is any doubt that wet is red hot, just look around you. Music videos are full of bikini-clad models dancing poolside. Advertisers sell soft drinks with images of bare-chested, sweat-drenched men. Countless movies titillate us with scenes of shower sex. This collective understanding of sex appeal feeds into the fantasies of people like Mary, 28, who describes what ultimately gets her in the mood: "I love to watch movies with shower scenes. I think it's because my first notion of sex came when I was watching one of my mom's soap operas with her. One of the main characters had sex in a shower, and I thought that was the most exciting thing ever. Something about that has held over, and now, every time I see a shower scene, I get really turned on."

Like Mary, forty-two-year-old Brian's favorite fantasy was triggered by something he saw years ago. "I just need to think about the scene in *Flashdance*, where Jennifer Beals dumps the water on her head after dancing on stage. That might just be the hottest thing I have ever seen. When I think about that scene, I get hard instantly."

For Lyle, 34, the image of a sweaty girl is turn-on enough. "When I masturbate, I imagine women dripping with sweat. Sometimes they are dressed in little tank tops or ripped white t-shirts, and sometimes they are totally naked and slick. When I have sex with a woman, I love to get her to that point. I like to have sex under the covers just so we can become totally wet with sweat. I also love having sex in the summer when it is so hot that even the smallest movement gets you dripping wet."

Sam, 29, dreams of one day living out her fantasy of going to a poolside orgy. "I'm really into the idea of a pool party turning into a sex-fest, with couples screwing in the water and girls walking around topless and wearing only tiny bikini bottoms."

Other common aquatic fantasies include frolicking nude on an isolated beach, having sex in a public pool, lathering up a lover under the shower, or being taken in a hot tub. Many people dream of being captured and ravished by pirates or becoming the plaything of a mysterious mermaid or virile sailor. Sometimes people worry that their fantasies are sick or perverse, but rest assured it is perfectly normal to have a rich and varied fantasy life. Here are a few things to keep in mind:

· Fantasies are perfectly normal and healthy.

· Sometimes people want to act out fantasies in real life, but often people are content to simply imagine certain acts, and would not be comfortable actually participating in them.

· Fantasies about being abused or degraded are not automatic reflections of real-life desires, and are not an indication that someone is twisted, mentally ill, or self-hating.

· Fantasizing is a healthy way to brainstorm ideas you may want to attempt in real life.

· Fantasizing while having sex play with a partner does not indicate a lack of satisfaction with that person. Rather, doing so can be a great way to spice up a sexual encounter.

· Sharing fantasies with a lover can be a sexy and rewarding experience, but not sharing fantasies is also perfectly fine. Fantasies can be our own sexy little secrets that we don't have to feel guilty about keeping.

· If you've never tried fantasizing before, give it a whirl! Find a time and place where you won't be bothered. Close your eyes and try to picture something that turns you on. Let a story or image evolve. Try not to censor or judge yourself for the places your mind might wander.

Sandra and Snow

"I had my first kiss in the snow. I was a teenager, and my friend Maggie and I were throwing snowballs at each other and running around my backyard having fun. At one point she tackled me and pinned my arms down. We just sat there for a while catching our breath. I could feel the snow soaking through my jeans and dripping down the back of my shirt, but I didn't really care. Then Maggie leaned over and kissed me. Not a peck either. She slipped her tongue in my mouth and gave me my first French kiss. We lay in the snow kissing for what seemed like hours and then went inside completely soaked and frozen. It was one of the most exciting experiences of my life, and one I have never been able to re-create. I like to think about that when I'm masturbating, and remember how it felt to lie frozen and wet on the ground while getting this extremely hot kiss."

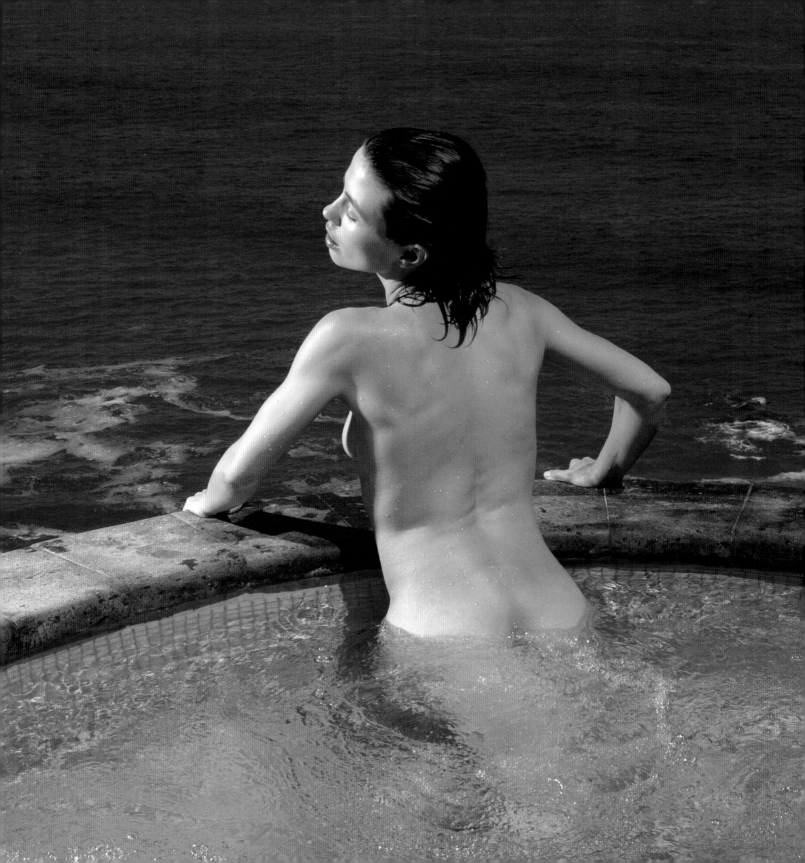

Solo Sloshing

There are countless ways that people incorporate water into their solo sessions. And the bathroom offers the perfect setting for self-exploration. Not only does the bathroom provide privacy, but a steamy shower or bath can get you worked into quite a lather. Women often take particular joy in the handheld shower nozzle. "My first orgasm was using my shower nozzle," says Aimee, 27. "I had tried to make myself come before, just using my hand, without much success. One day I was in the shower and I put the nozzle between my legs. The next thing I knew I was feeling these waves of pleasure wash over me. I can come in other ways now, but I love to make myself come that way—it's so reliable and sexy."

Ariella, 22, also mastered the running water trick. However, she did so in the tub. "I love to take baths. I fill the tub half way. I light candles and turn off the lights and use plenty of bubble bath. I don't let the water get too high at first. Then I get in and scoot under the running faucet and lie back with my legs up. I have a bath pillow, which makes it really comfortable. This is actually the best way for me to come, and afterward I can just soak in the tub as long as I like."

Gabrielle, 28, isn't a shower enthusiast, but she loves to touch herself outside by her pool. "One of my favorite things to do is to lay out by my pool in a little bikini. I'll usually take off my top and play with myself under my bottoms. I always hope that someone will look over the fence and see me, or that my husband will come home and catch me. It hasn't happened yet, but there are still plenty of sunny days left."

On the other end of the spectrum is Adam, 23, who explains, "Rain turns me on. I love to lie in bed masturbating when it's raining. It's like I have an excuse to stay in bed and jack-off all day without feeling bad about not being outside in the good weather."

One of the best ways to get yourself off is to figure out what gets you hot. Sexual arousal is all about desire. Often this desire is directed at a specific person, but it can also be focused on a situation, an object, or a physical sensation. Though many people can clearly tell you what they find arousing, others might need to really think long and hard before being able to identify their turn-ons. To do so you might want to ask yourself the following questions:

· What was I doing the last time I got aroused?

· What movie scene do I find sexiest?

· If I imagine myself having sex, where am I?

· What types of sex acts turn me on? Kissing? Body rubbing? Oral? Anal? Straight-up screwing?

· What part of a person's body do I find most appealing?

· What is sexier: being naked or wearing clothing?

· Do I get excited thinking about:

Having sex in public?

Being tied up?

Being spanked?

Having sex in the water?

Having sex with more than one person?

Wearing or having my partner wear lingerie?

Watching porn?

Going to a strip club?

A romantic bubble bath with a lover?

There are many other questions you might want to ask yourself when trying to figure out your turn-ons, but starting with these is a great step toward discovering even your most hidden desires.

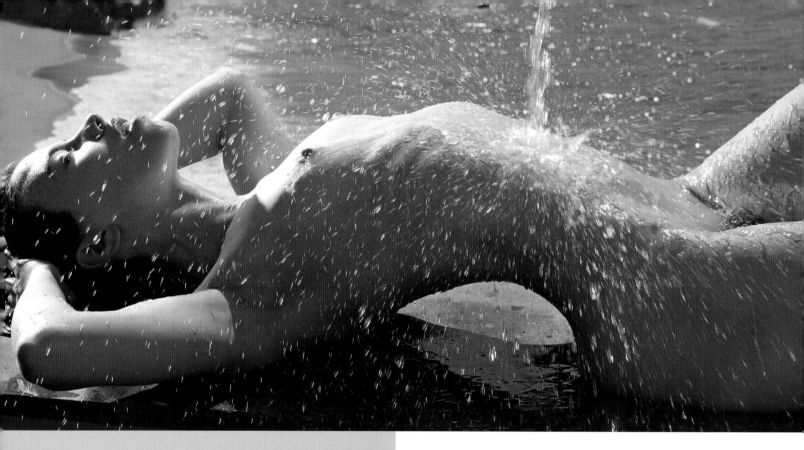

Desmond's Hot Spots

"For a long time I was worried that I was abnormal because I didn't get turned on by things other guys were into. Pamela Anderson doesn't do it for me, and I could care less about the Victoria's Secret catalogue or watching porn. I just thought I had a low sex drive. But a few years ago, I went to a burlesque show with some friends. One of the acts was a really curvy girl wearing a latex dress and patent leather shoes. Part of her performance included being sprayed by a hose so she was completely glistening and wet. The water just made the latex seem even more formfitting and slick and clean. I got really turned on, and ever since then I've used that image to help me get hard. I've even come up with a few variations on the scene, most of which involve me spraying her and then peeling off her clothes. I wouldn't say I have a fetish, but now I definitely have something I can tap into if I am trying to get aroused."

So How Do I Sail Solo?

It is perfectly normal and healthy for both men and women to masturbate, whether they are single or in a relationship. Masturbation is safe and fun, and it is a great way to learn about your body and relieve stress. Unfortunately, however, many people are uncomfortable masturbating. We are told that men who masturbate are the equivalent of sex-starved teenagers, and plenty of women have heard that "nice girls don't masterbate." Well, I am here to tell you plenty of nice (and naughty) girls and guys do! Accepting that it's normal to masturbate is the crucial first step. The second is actually peeling off your underwear and going for it.

Solo Sailing for Ladies

Follow the steps below for some serious solo-sailing:

1. Find a private place where you won't be disturbed.

2. Get comfy.

3. Set the mood. Think of a hot sailor taking you under the dock, watch porn, or read something super-sexy.

4. Don't just dive between your legs, stroke the rest of your body, touch your breasts, and let yourself relax.

5. Now that you're relaxed and aroused, start exploring your pink parts.

6. Hold your labia apart and draw some of your natural juices up your vulva. If you aren't that wet, try using some Astroglide or Wet lube.

7. Now, find your clitoris.

8. Roll your clit between your fingers. Figure out whether it is more comfortable to do this using your labia for pressure, or whether you prefer the direct touch of your fingers.

9. While rubbing your clitoris, try sliding your fingers into your vagina. See how many are comfortable. Does it feel better to hold them there, or to slide them in and out of your body?

10. If you like G-spot stimulation, use a toy or your finger to try to locate this area.

11. Add a vibrator. Position it on your clitoris, or anywhere else that feels good. You may be surprised at how quickly you can come or how intense the orgasm can be. Try experimenting with a G-spot vibrator.

12. Try a few different positions to see what feels best.

For a super-hot (and educational) video on female masturbation, check out *Betty Dodson's Orgasmic Woman: 13 Self-Loving Divas.*

WET 'N WILD

Fill a plastic bag with ice cubes. Rub the bag of ice cubes around your nipples and other places you like to feel sensation, then move down to your vulva. Draw the bag over your clit and feel tingling sensations dance across your entire body!

Solo Sailing for the Fellas

There is a general assumption that all men know how to make themselves climax in no time flat. While this is the case for plenty of guys, it this isn't a universal truth. Some men have difficulties making themselves come. Like women with the same issue, men need to accept that masturbation is perfectly healthy and normal. Once they do, the technical aspects will be much more likely to fall into place. Fantasizing, focusing on sensation, and practicing a variety of techniques can be helpful.

Meanwhile, men who don't have a problem reaching orgasm may become bored with their preferred method of doing so. A lot of men masturbate by wrapping their fingers around their hard penis and stroking it up and down until they climax. This tried-and-true method works wonderfully for many fellas, but that doesn't mean there isn't room for variation or improvement. Stimulating other areas, such as the testicles, anus, prostate, inner thighs, or nipples while stroking your penis can enhance the masturbatory experience.

Here are some additional techniques that can change up your usual routine:

• Circle your penis with your thumb and forefinger, and stroke up and down your shaft. When you get to the top, close your fingers in a circle, then squeeze as you slide back down to the bottom of your shaft.

• With one hand, stroke your penis from top to the bottom. When you reach the base, release your grip. Switch hands repeatedly and develop a rhythm.

• Push your penis into your closed fist as though you were penetrating it. Change hands and repeat the motion.

• Only touch your shaft, avoiding the head. Keep this up for as long as possible before letting yourself touch the head softly with your fingers.

• While stroking your penis, insert a butt plug for added anal sensation or prostate stimulation.

For the most comprehensive information about male masturbation on the Internet, check out www.jackinworld.com.

WET 'N WILD

If you're the kind of guy who likes to get off in the shower, avoid using shampoo or soap as a lube, as it can get into the urethra and burn! Try an artificial lube for a smoother sail.

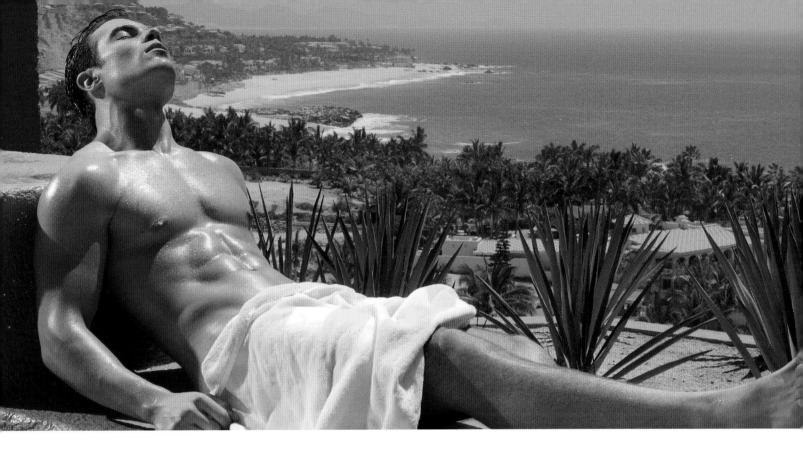

The Best Solo-Sailing Spots

Now that you are an expert at self-love, try experimenting with a few hot spots for a session. There are plenty of good wet options. As I mentioned, the shower, tub, and poolside are common venues. Here are some other locations you can consider for solo sex play:

· Hot tubs

· Saunas

· A secluded beach

· A public beach

· The ocean

· Your backyard under the sprinkler

· Your front yard under the sprinkler

· Beside a forest or mountain stream

· The dock on a lake

· A raft, canoe, or sailboat

· Under or next to a waterfall

Picking the perfect spot can turn your sex play in to a ride of wet and wonderful pleasure, and one you'll be using as fantasy fodder for years to come. While many people get turned on by particularly nautical venues, others simply like the idea of getting caught in the act. If this is your thing, keep in mind, the fantasy might be more exciting than the reality. Many people would be quite put-off to stumble across a solo stroker, and the results of such a meeting could be far from the fantasy you envision!

WET 'N WILD

Remember this is all about you! For the hottest solo sessions, find a time when you won't be disturbed. There is no need to rush or worry about how you look or sound. Use your solo time to try out things you might not be completely ready to do with a partner.

> "*Masturbation* is our first natural sexual activity . . . Masturbation is a way to gain *sexual self-knowledge*. Cultural denial of masturbation is the basis of sexual repression. Sharing masturbation with a lover enhances *sexual intimacy*. Being responsible for our own orgasm gives us a choice when it comes to *partner sex*."
>
> —Betty Dodson, *Sex for One*

Show Him How It's Done!

Now that you are an expert at self-love, it is time to let your honey in on the secret. Many people are shy about showing someone how they come. At best, masturbation is thought of as something to be done in private; at worst, it is seen as a perversion. Nevertheless, watching a partner get him- or herself off can be one of the hottest and most intimate experiences a couple can share. It is also a great way to learn about a lover's turn-ons and techniques. Mark, 31, explains that the shower was the first place he felt comfortable demonstrating to his partner how to make him come. "I have a pretty specific way I like to have my member held. I was a little shy asking my girlfriend to do that. But we took a shower together, and as she was soaping me up, I started to get hard. She went for my penis, but I kind of stopped her, and asked if I could show her what I do. She was really into it, and saw how I liked to be touched without me having to tell her she had been doing anything wrong."

Here are a few other ways to show your lover how to please you:

· Be direct! Try saying things like, "a little harder," "that feels great, now try moving a bit to the left," and "I love how you touch me. It would be really exciting to also feel you touching me like this . . ."

· If you don't want to use words, try actions. Gently move a partner's hand or mouth. Change positions to one that is more comfortable for you. Grab a bottle of lube and pass it over.

· Make it a game. Tell your sweetie that you are going to put on a special show for his or her eyes only. If you want to get saucy, hand over a pen and paper and give instructions to take copious notes. Then work yourself into an orgasmic frenzy, explaining what you are doing as you go.

Not everyone instantly meshes in bed. This isn't a character flaw. Nor does it mean you are destined for a life of bad sex. Failing to satisfy a lover can be a blow to the sexual ego, but a good lover will try to solve the problem and work through it. So be open to showing a lover how you come, or letting a lover show you how he or she gets off. Solo-sailing may start out as a one-handed job, but there is no reason it has to stay that way.

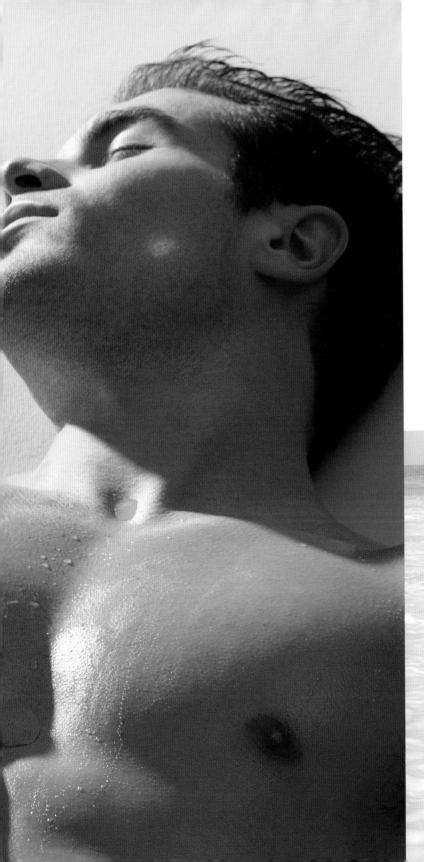

Romance for One

A romantic vacation does not have to be something you only enjoy with a lover. Getting away by yourself to a tropical hot spot or wintry paradise can be a great time for relaxation and self-exploration, of both the sexual and emotional variety. Check yourself into a luxurious spa or seaside resort and enjoy pampering to the fullest without any concern for another person's needs. Enjoy massages, take long saunas, refresh yourself with dips in the pool, then relax with a chilled cocktail overlooking the ocean before turning in for the day and treating yourself to the type of orgasm only you know how to provide. Far from being lonely, you'll discover just how nice it is to enjoy quality alone time.

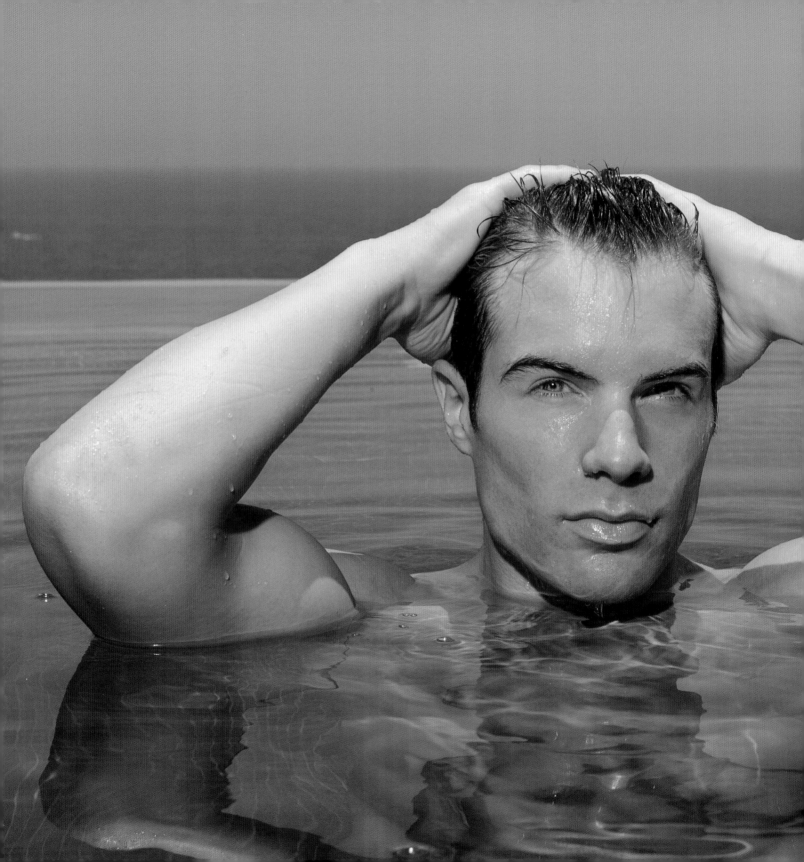

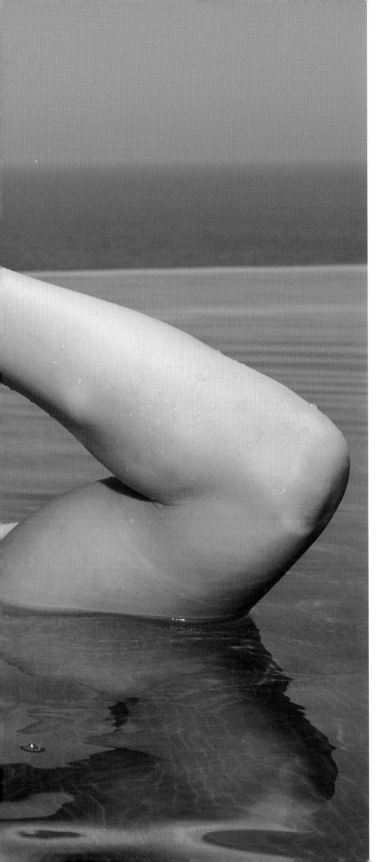

We live in a culture that idealizes couples. Single folks are often made to feel there is something wrong with them for not being paired up. Similarly, self-sexual exploration is often seen as distasteful or pathetic. These unfortunate beliefs cause a lot of needless grief and self-doubt. It is crucial to acknowledge that it is perfectly acceptable to explore your sexual side, whether you are single or part of a couple. Once you can embrace this notion, you will be able to explore your body and your desires, and conquer fears and barriers that might have been holding you back from a sizzling sex life.

Looking to water for sensual inspiration can help you discover your sexiest side. Try out as many watery venues as you can think of; slosh around in the tub, break out a vibrator, watch some mermaid porn, or just tune into the wettest fantasies your imagination can come up with. Share your newfound discoveries with a lover or keep them to yourself. Whatever you do, if you make getting to know your body intimately a priority, your sex life will most definitely thank you!

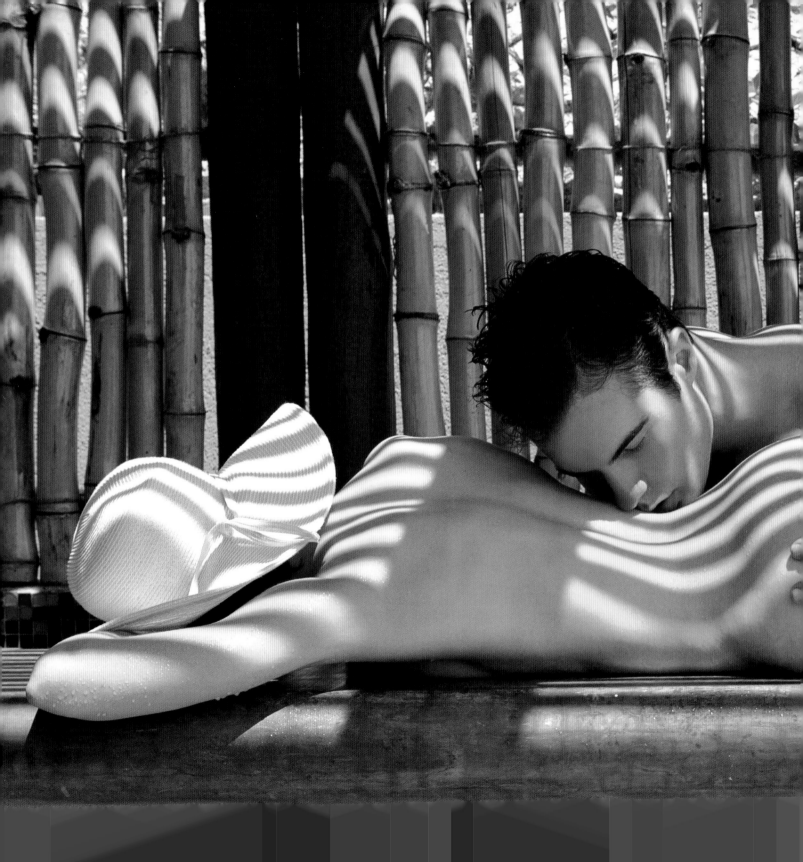

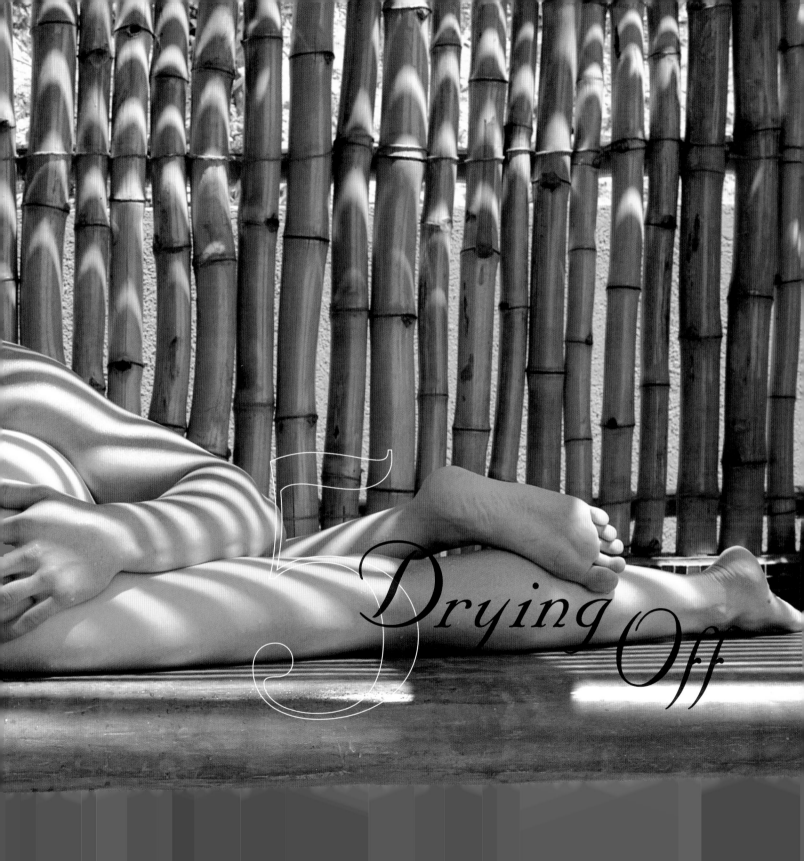

Drying Off

5 Drying Off

WATER IS CRUCIAL TO OUR SURVIVAL. It makes up more than 70 percent of the human body, cleans and sustains us better than any other substance, and of course, offers countless erotic opportunities. Throughout history, humans have identified the connection between water and sensuality, so it is not surprising that this life-giving element appeals to so many of our most basic instincts.

Wet Looks

Plenty of us are visual creatures who enjoy feasting our eyes on the objects of our desire. You might have heard that men become aroused by what they see, while women's arousal is connected to what they hear. In reality, this just isn't the case. People of both sexes find their hearts racing and their loins throbbing when they glimpse at something sexually appealing. Though everyone finds different things arousing, plenty of people agree that seeing the wet, slick body of someone they wouldn't mind rolling around with naked ranks pretty high on the list. There is an easy explanation for this. Wet bodies look sexier than dry ones. Skin, moist with water, sweat, and even suntan oil, shimmers and catches light in a sensual manner. Wet clothes highlight contours only partially hidden underneath. Even the sight of a sexy figure lounging luxuriously next to a body of water can be erotic fantasy fodder. Wetness captures and conveys sexuality better than any other element, teasing and delighting the eye and triggering the body's natural responses.

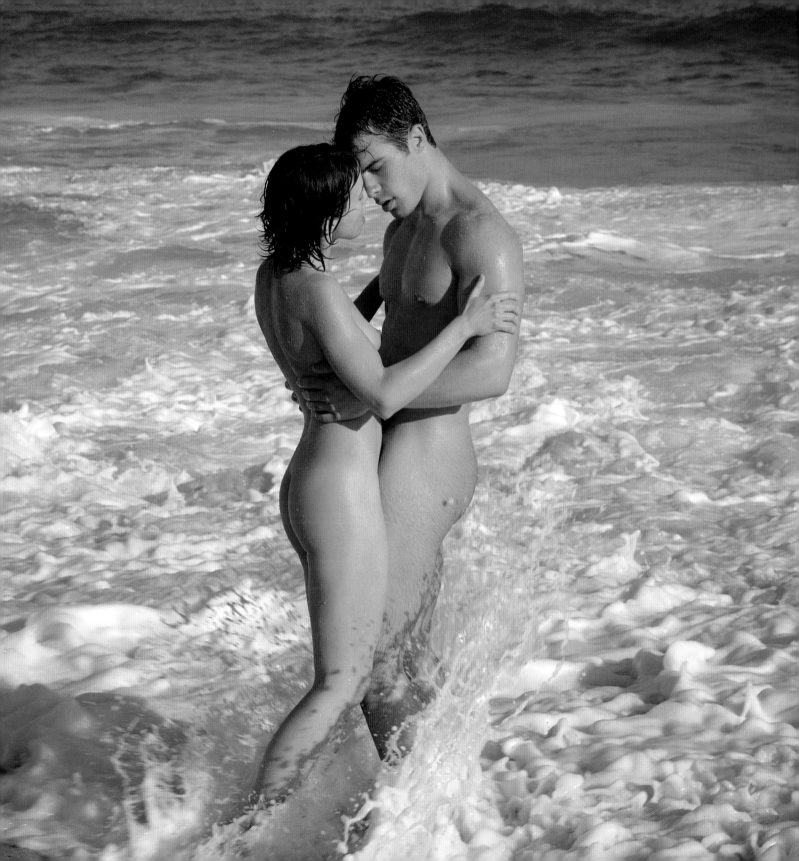

Wet Sensations

Nothing feels better than a relaxing soak in the tub, a hot shower after a long day, or an invigorating swim in a sparkling pool. Submerging yourself in a body of water is a treat for all your senses. Water can be sensual, soothing, or bracing. Warm water envelopes the body in a cocoon of comfort, while the cold stuff forces you into heightened alertness of a different variety. Sex play in the water adds sensation to an already tactile experience. Being bathed by a lover, having ice run slowly over your tingling flesh, or giving in to the powers of a delectable liquid massage can bring your body awareness to heights previously unknown. Combining a lover's caress with the warmth of water engulfing your entire body will make you wonder why there is any need for dry land whatsoever.

Wet Tastes

Thirst is a terrible feeling that gnaws at our throats and fills us with an aching need for relief. In fact, quenching your thirst may be one of the most physically rewarding experiences imaginable. Drinking down a cool beverage, sipping at a cocktail, or even enjoying your morning tea are all things we take for granted. But drinking is not just about sustenance. It can also be a sensually delicious experience in and of itself—especially when what we are drinking is our lover's body. Tasting your lover's fluids can be an intrinsic part of a sexual union. Drinking up a lover's juices or licking the sweat from his navel or from the furrow between her breasts can invite a connection not experienced when sex play is kept neat and tidy. To taste someone is to truly know them in the deepest way possible. How our bodies taste reflect our very essence, and while we often try to mask these with scents and soaps, the act of truly savoring another person's core being is possibly the most intimate act two individuals can share.

Wet Sounds

Of all the romantic settings, there are few places that rival the water's edge. The lapping of waves against the shore creates a sense of serenity and peacefulness that many people enjoy quietly sharing with a lover. But our ears do not only have to be soothed to feel sensual. Many people desire aural sounds of a much less delicate nature. If you fall into this camp, try incorporating your appreciation for aquatics into your dirty talk. Explain all the wet ways you are about to take your lover. Whisper that you want to wash him from head to toe or lick honey from her thighs. Break out the porn and pick a sexy story from one of the many aquatic erotica collections available. Then crawl between the sheets and take turns thrilling each other's ears with your wettest words.

Wet Games

Sex is supposed to be fun and exciting, so what better way to make it so than by adding water? Wet sex offers up possibilities that are remarkably creative yet simple to execute. You can spontaneously splash around in your tub, make passionate love on a secluded beach, or spritz your honey with a hose. Or you can plan out a more involved encounter and use props to assume a nighttime nautical identity for a hot role play. Even childhood games like Hide and Seek, Simon Says, and Mother May I can be turned into sexy water adventures with just a little creativity and imagination.

"*My wife* and I were working in our garden one day—she was planting flowers and I was watering them—and I decided to spray her *just for fun.* She started to try to wrestle the hose away from me, and we both ended up drenched. At one point we were on the ground, wrestling, and I became *extremely turned on.* There was something *incredibly primal* about both of us being sopping wet and muddy, that I had to take her right there. Luckily we have a fence around our backyard, so none of our neighbors could see us. The hose came in particularly handy when I was *pleasuring my wife!*"

—Daniel, 36

Wet Spots

We all know that when shopping for real estate, location is everything. Location is also a key factor to consider when shopping for sizzling sex spots. Whether you are envisioning beach romance, a quickie in the neighbor's hot tub, or a luxurious bath *à deux*, the place you choose for your aquatic adventure can be almost as important as the physical experience itself. When thinking about a setting, consider a few things:

- Does it turn me on?
- Will my partner be comfortable there?
- Am I looking for complete privacy, or do I want to explore a little exhibitionism?
- Is it safe (and legal)?
- Will I need props?
- Do I need to scout it out first?

Asking these questions before your encounter, and not in the middle of it, will make the entire experience a much smoother sail.

Wet Moves

We've all looked through sex manuals boasting positions with improbable names that require impossible feats of athleticism and wondered, "Who can actually do *that*?" In some cases the answer is: "No one." In others it is: "You, with a little help from the wet stuff." Using water as a prop can facilitate positions that might otherwise require great strength or acrobatic training. Water is buoyant and can help maneuver you into poses and contortions that just wouldn't be possible on dry land. Once you are surrounded by water, you and your partner will experience weightlessness and flexibility that just isn't possible in bed.

Additionally, the freedom you will feel in the midst of a vast body of water will allow for exploration and sexual discovery. Plenty of kids thrill themselves by doing underwater somersaults and handstands—isn't it time that adults took advantage of abilities that only come out when completely submerged?

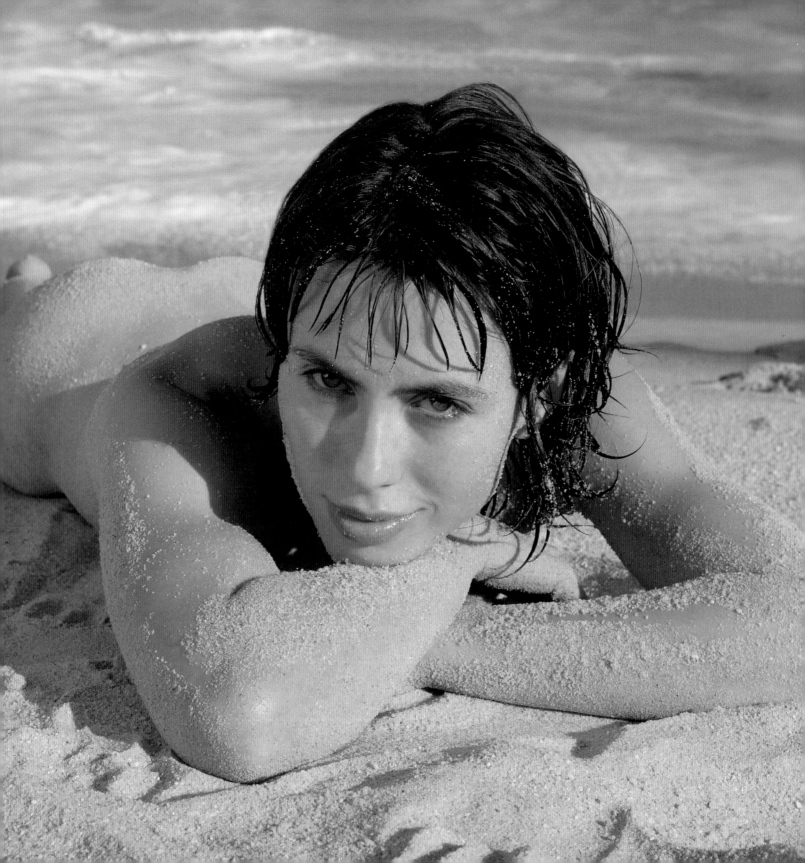

The Wet-list

The beauty of wet sex is that there are so many different places for it to occur. Props and supplies can enhance sex play and facilitate a greater variety of activities. So follow the sound advice of the Boy Scouts and "be [situationally] prepared" for your wet ride.

The Tub

The first thing you need for a sensual soak is a tub, preferably large and sparkling clean. Then apply ample bubble bath, dribble in scented essential oils or add flower petals, and set the mood by lowering the lights and lighting candles. Whether you are soaking alone or with your lover, erotica and porn can be a welcome addition. If you aren't planning on moving around excessively, you might want to opt for floating candles. If you are planning on shifting from bathtub romance to straight-up sex, use well-placed bath pillows to maximize comfort and prevent bruised knees or elbows. For more playful bathtub sessions, throw in toys (either the waterproof sex-toy variety or those specifically designed for kids). Bring a spray bottle, waterproof finger-paints, and plenty of sponges for squeezing, washing, and sudsing up your sweetie.

The Shower

Mood plays a big role in the bathroom. Decide what mood you are going for and then set the stage. Sometimes all you need to kick start shower sex is a transparent shower curtain so that your honey can play the voyeur, or you the exhibitionist. However, the most versatile shower prop of all is the handheld shower nozzle. This innocent device has probably been responsible for more orgasms than store-bought vibrators, and it is a great tool for sexy shower play with a partner.

The Beach

Towels, bug spray, and sunscreen might not seem like the sexiest supplies to accompany a romantic encounter. However, if you are going for it out in the elements, trust me, having these few basics will let you concentrate on the hot session in the sand, and not on the mosquitoes stinging your most intimate places. Similarly, a well-positioned umbrella and a big beach blanket can mean the difference between multiple orgasms and receiving a summons for public sex!

The Pool

If you are planning on playing underwater games with your honey, make sure you bring any necessary supplies. These might include a blindfold, blowup raft, or easily removable bathing suit. Sturdy and comfortable lounge chairs, pillows, and suntan oil can further enhance poolside encounters. The supplies you need will likely be slightly different depending on whether you are diving into a private oasis, or meeting up with your honey amidst the sweaty throngs crowding a community pool on a hot summer day. Though some folks get off on the spontaneity and surprise of unplanned sex, preparation can play a part in getting you hot.

The Hot Tub

The hot tub requires fewer props than most venues, seeing as it comes equipped with all those handy jets! Still you might want to bring along a waterproof pillow and create a romantic atmosphere with candles and music. The hot tub is a great place to indulge your taste buds. Mix up a batch of margaritas or mojitos. Sip your favorite wine or champagne. Try a cold drink to contrast the hot water and experience the different sensations coursing through your body.

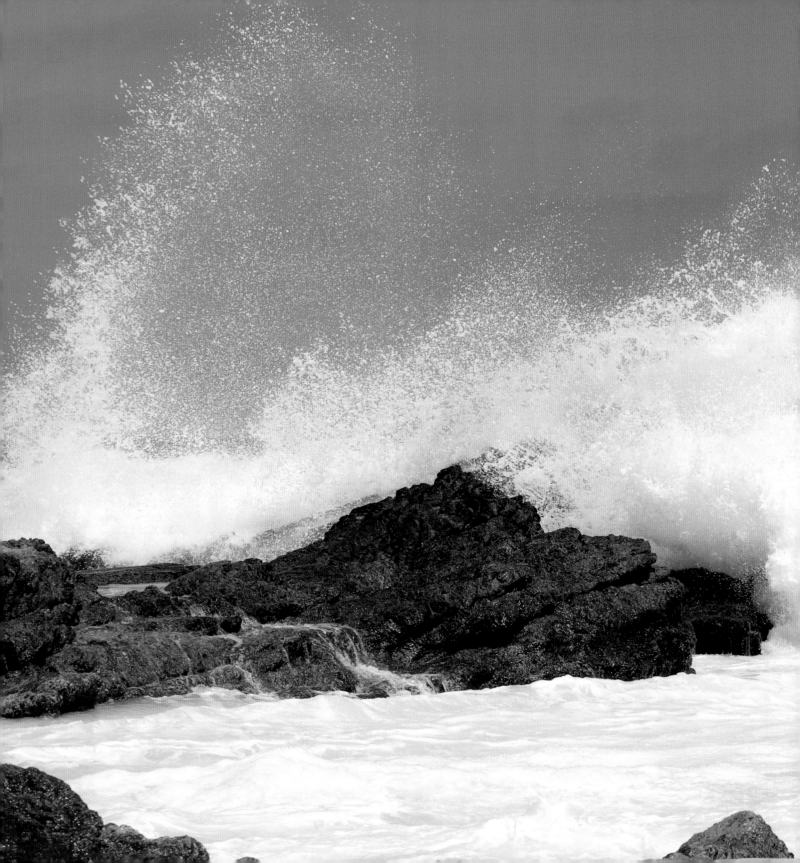

The Bedroom

Though not an aquatic location on its own, the bedroom lends itself to wet play in a variety of ways. Slip into costume to act out naughty nautical fantasies, or use your lover's body as a canvas for your body paint and liquid latex creations. See what response a little ice can elicit. Coat your sweetie in chocolate sauce, whipped cream, or honey, and then lick her clean. Find out what your favorite liqueur tastes like off his body.

The bedroom is also a great place for a massage. Use a massage oil you like or make your own with safflower, grapeseed, or sweet almond oil scented with rosehip seed oil, lemongrass essential oil, or vanilla oil. Make sure that your hands are warm before you start and then treat your honey to full body work-over.

Wet Sex Play Anywhere

Lube is essential to sex play. Lubricants enhance sensation, and make sex more pleasurable, slippery, and safe. Try out a few different brands to see which work for you. Remember, when having sex in the water, use a waterproof silicone lube to make up for the fact that a woman's natural vaginal lubrication will likely get washed away. If you are practicing safer sex, keep condoms in a handy place where you can easily find them. But don't keep them for too long. Just like milk, latex comes with an expiration date!

Bringing It Up with Your Honey

So how do you tell your honey you want to move things from the boudoir to the shower, or that your ideal vacation involves private hot tub lovemaking sessions, or that you have a penchant for messy wrestling? What words can you use to explain your sailor fantasy, or why you find wet t-shirt contests so appealing? Our sexual desires can be hard to discuss, and many people clam up when they need to vocalize their desires. If you are finding talking tough, try writing.

You and your lover should each compile a list of sexy activities that you would like to do together. Switch lists and make three categories. These can include: Things I'd like to try, Things I would consider trying, and Things I never want to try. Your partner may have never considered having sex on a diving board or watching mermaid porn, but it might not sound so bad when you discuss the possibilities. That said, another person might balk at the idea of making love on a public beach, and that's okay too. Discussing our desires is not the same thing as pressuring an uncomfortable partner into doing something he or she just doesn't find appealing There are so many ways to explore our sexuality that once you each come up with a solid list, you are bound to find aqueous activities that appeal to you both!

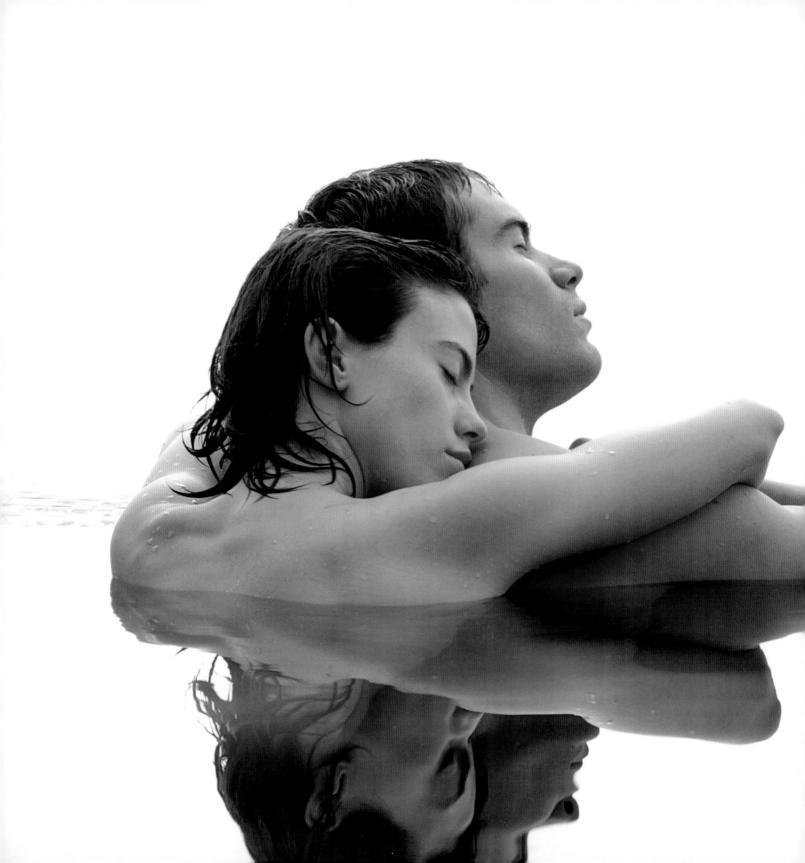

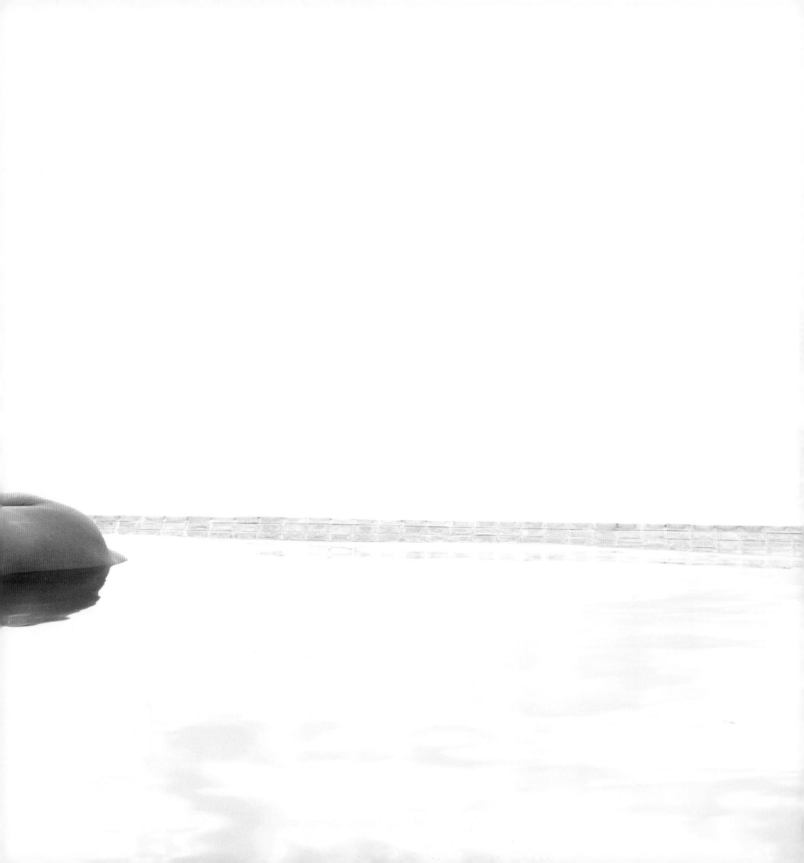

It's a Wash

Soothing, searing, seductive, scorching or sensual—make sex play wet, and you never know what kind of experience you will have! Aqueous encounters offer countless possibilities for expression and adventure. They can be romantic, naughty, or just plain fun. Whether you are splashing around in your tub or making passionate love under a crashing waterfall, there's no denying the power of water. Still skeptical? Next time it rains, forget the umbrella. Step outside and get soaked to the bone. Then imagine all the ways water can do more than just drench you, because as you now know, getting wet is just that much more sensual, sexy, and life affirming than staying dry!

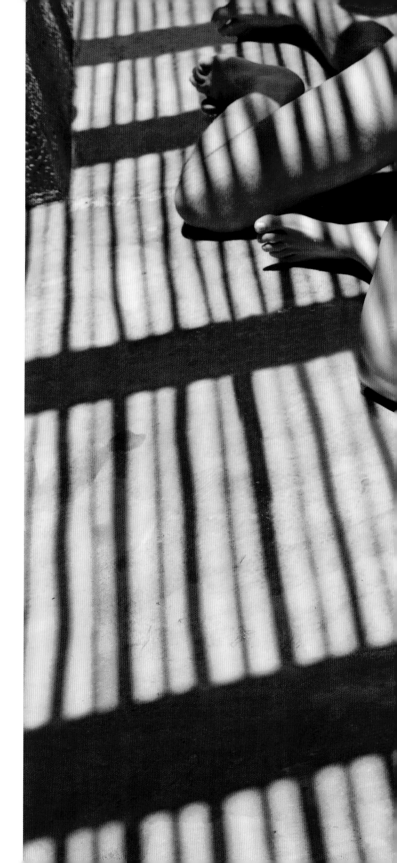

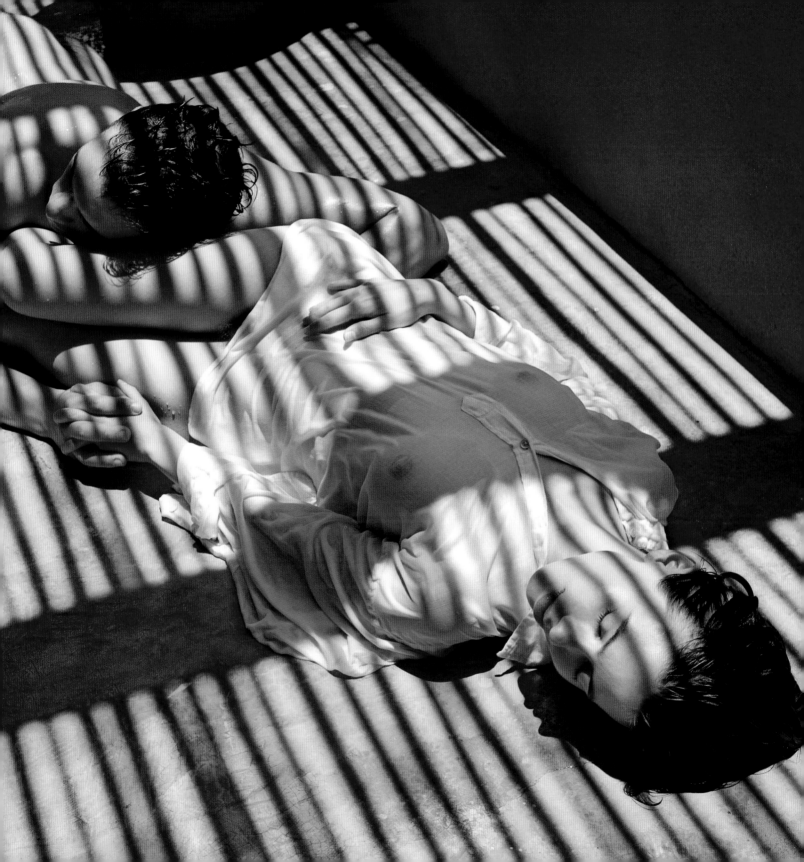

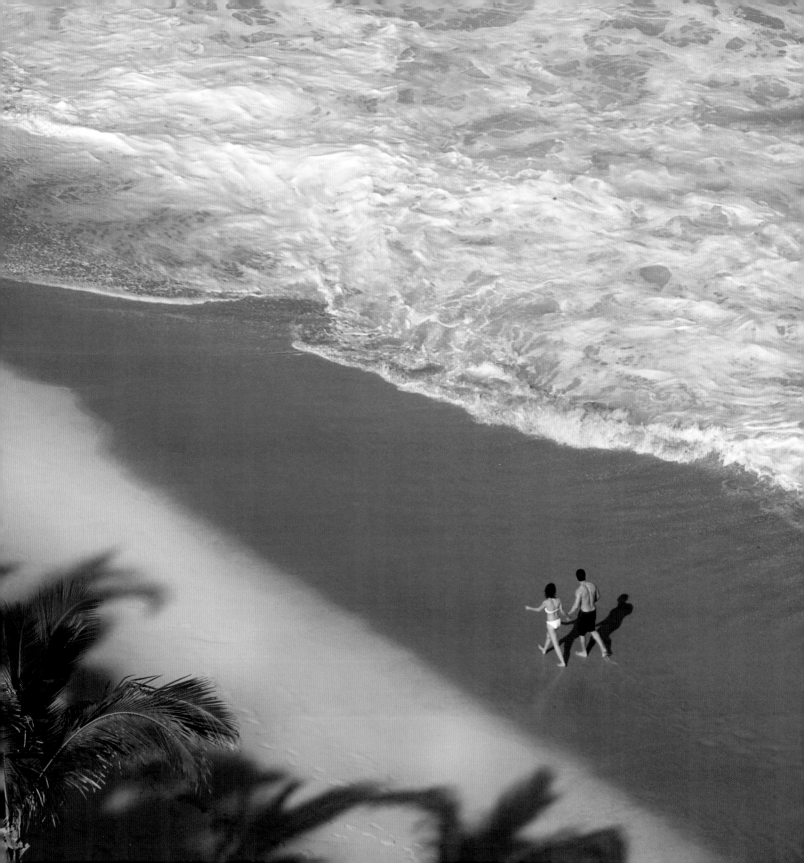

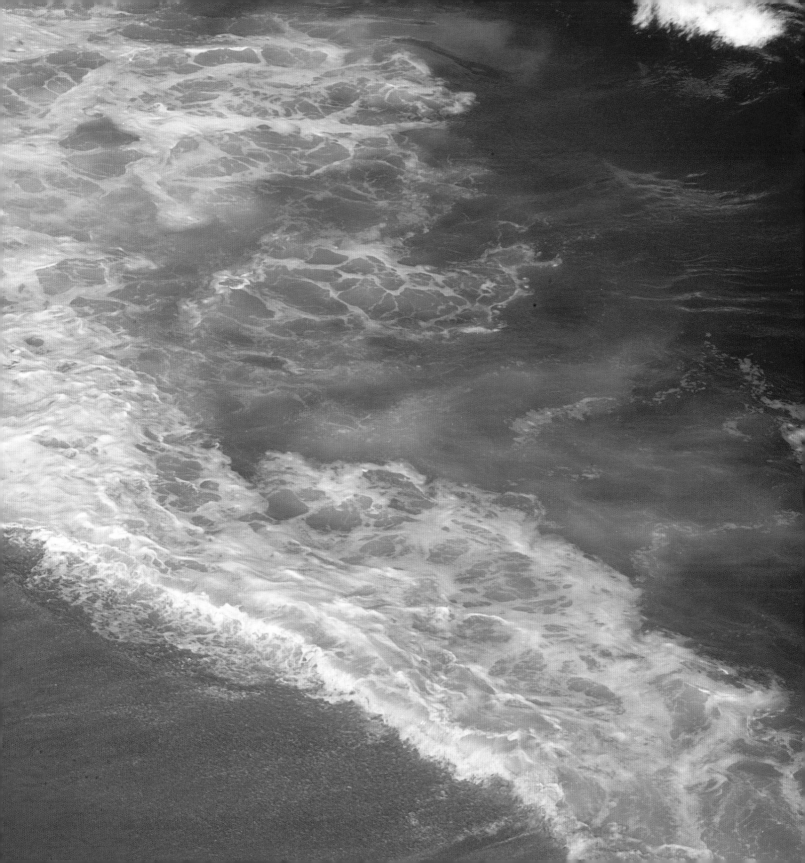

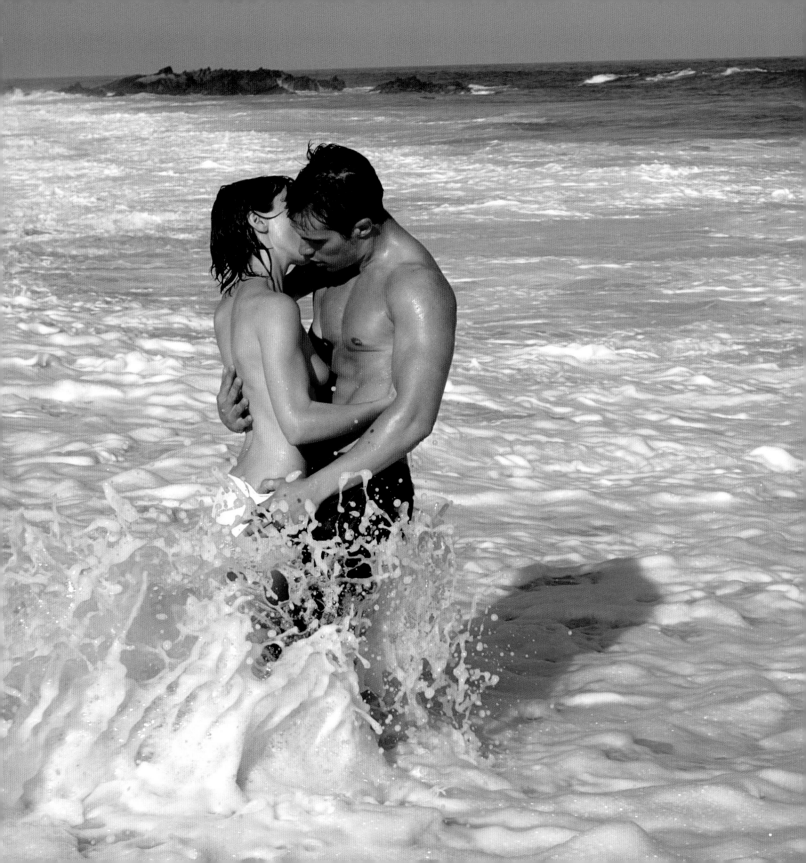

ABOUT THE AUTHOR

ELLEN KATE is a sexuality educator who holds a MA in health and human sexuality education from New York University. She was previously the Director of Public Programs at the Museum of Sex in New York City. She currently teaches college human sexuality classes and runs workshops on topics such as achieving orgasm, sex toys, and sexy, safer sex. She lives in Brooklyn, New York.

OTHER HOT BOOKS FROM QUIVER

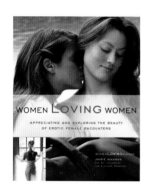

Women Loving Women
Appreciating and Exploring the Beauty of Erotic Female Encounters
By Jamye Waxman

ISBN-13: 978-159233-258-8
ISBN-10: 1-59233-258-7
$19.99/£12.99/$25.95 CAN

Women Loving Women explores the phenomenon of the contemporary "bi-sexual" or "lesbian" experience for the heterosexual woman and simultaneously places this age-old obsession in a historical perspective. The book also responds to how same-sex encounters might actually spice up a woman's heterosexual relationship (as many men fantasize about same-sex women encounters), break the ice with a best friend, or simply add a new dimension to her sexual history. Testimonials from heterosexual women who have experienced same-sex romantic encounters are featured throughout. Sidebars also feature stories of women-who-have-loved-women throughout history, such as Virginia Woolf and Eleanor Roosevelt, amongst others.

The photographs, shot on location in New Hampshire, tell the story of three beautiful women who leave their boyfriends/husbands behind for a "girls weekend" and discover a new dimension to their friendship.

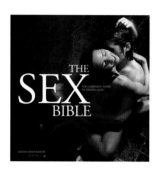

The Sex Bible
The Complete Guide to Sexual Love
By Susan Crain Bakos

ISBN-13: 978-1-59233-227-4
ISBN-10: 1-59233-227-7
$30.00/£19.99/$38.95 CAN

The Sex Bible is an authoritative, comprehensive, and beautifully photographed sex resource that provides in-depth treatment of sexual topics in frank detail. The book is arranged into different sections, including "Foreplay," "Sex Toys," and "Oral Sex." It explores sexual subjects you are either familiar with, or until now, never even knew existed. Couples will be captivated by personal anecdotes interspersed throughout. Illustrated with full-color photography, *The Sex Bible* will not only educate couples, but also it will help heighten sexual enjoyment.

www.quiverbooks.com

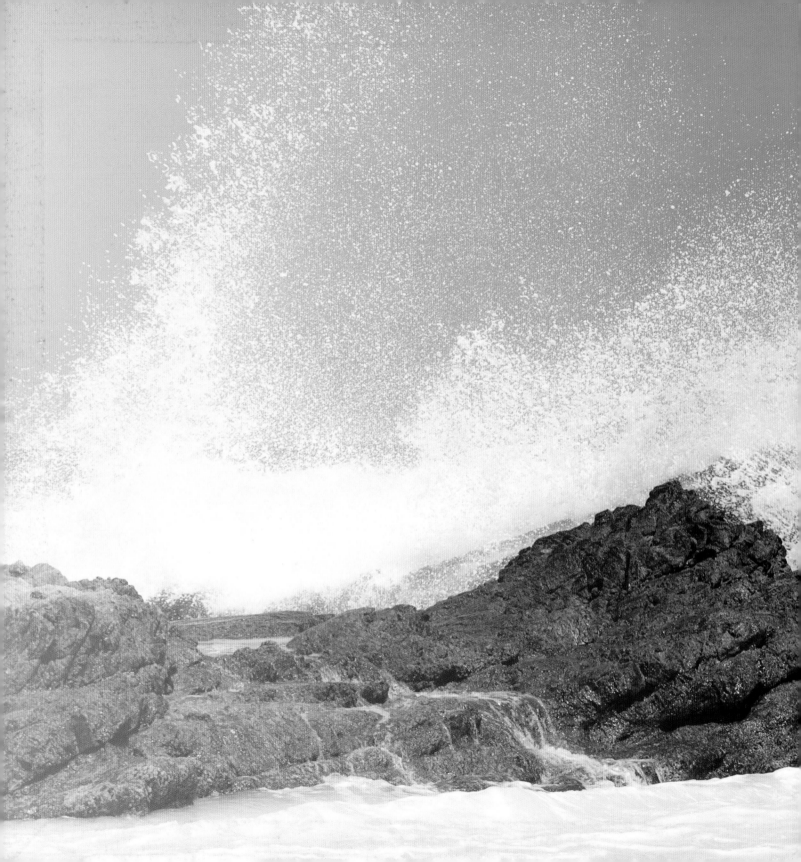